"This is not just another book on a trendy medical topic. Dr. Rosemarie Moser is a passionate clinician whose extensive experience with sports-related concussions caused me to dramatically change my own methods for evaluation and treatment. Having the opportunity to work and engage in public forums side by side with her has given me a firsthand view of how much the public needs to be made aware of this topic. It is only fitting that she be the one to pen this text."

> —G. Luke Hensel, MSSM, ATC, LAT, SCC, head athletic trainer, Princeton Day School, and professional player and head athletic trainer, BuxMont Torch F.C., National Premier Soccer League

"We are very fortunate to have Dr. Moser as our team's concussion doctor. She truly understands our players and how to protect their brains. I commend her for creating this guidebook that will help protect the brains of our young athletes."

> —Ron Jaworski, co-owner, Philadelphia Soul Arena professional football team, ESPN Monday Night Football commentator, former Philadelphia Eagles NFL quarterback, and author of *The Games That Changed the Game: The Evolution of the NFL in Seven Sundays*

"As the medical director and school physician for a private boarding high school over the last 18 years, I have broad experience managing concussions in the adolescent population and have spent many hours caring for and educating students, coaches, athletic training staff, school nurses, faculty/teachers, and parents about concussions. I especially believe that educating parents of young athletes is extremely important and will go a long way towards preventing catastrophic outcomes that we see so much in the news today. That is why Dr. Moser's book is so important and valuable for parents."

> —Robin S. Karpf, M.D., medical director, The Lawrenceville School

"I am honored to be included in this guidebook on sports concussion in kids, and I commend Dr. Moser on her efforts to educate the public."

> —U.S. Representative Bill Pascrell Jr., co-chair, Congressional Brain Injury Task Force

"Dr. Moser brings her decades of experience as a clinician, as a researcher, and most importantly, as a parent, to the forefront, in order to help others understand and manage this most perplexing and elusive injury. If your child is playing sports at any level, this book is a must-read for you, as well as your child's coach and physician."

> —Philip Schatz, Ph.D., professor of psychology, St. Joseph's University

"Dr. Moser's helpful book discusses the process of managing sports-related concussions within the context of younger participants in sports, and focuses on fostering consensus around a child or adolescent's best interests and their well-being through cross-disciplinary teamwork. I recommend this excellent presentation and discussion on sports-related concussion for any parent who has many more questions than answers about the role of concussions in sports."

—Eric Zillmer, Psy.D., director of athletics and professor of neuropsychology, Drexel University, and author of *Principles of Neuropsychology*

"Dr. Moser takes her extensive clinical and research experience into the living room to give parents the nitty-gritty information they need to understand the current flap over sports-related concussions. Dr. Moser explains what concussions are, how they can affect the developing brains of children, how to facilitate recovery from concussions, and how to know that your concussed child is ready to return to activity. For parents, the news reports of athletes who suffer serious outcomes after concussions in sports raise questions about whether their children should risk playing some sports. Dr. Moser explains how risk can be evaluated and minimized, but also describes the red flags to look for in unsupervised leagues and youth sports. She tells parents how they can become involved in their communities to protect their children and keep the fun and 'play' in sports."

—Frank M. Webbe, Ph.D., professor of psychology and faculty athletics representative, Florida Institute of Technology, and author of *Handbook of Sports Neuropsychology*

"Once the occurrence of concussions in sports was not considered serious. Within recent years the issue of youth sports-related concussions has become a hot-button topic as there has been very strong evidence in the medical community that concussions left undiagnosed and untreated could have a far-reaching impact on families. In *Ahead of the Game*, Dr. Moser successfully takes on the mission to educate and share her experience and knowledge as a neuropsychologist, researcher, and sports mom to help other parents understand the critical importance of keeping kids' brains safe."

—Harry Carson, Pro Football Hall of Fame, former New York Giants NFL linebacker, and author of *Captain for Life: My Story as a Hall of Fame Linebacker*

AHEAD OF THE GAME

AHEAD OF THE GAME

THE PARENTS' GUIDE TO YOUTH SPORTS CONCUSSION

ROSEMARIE SCOLARO MOSER, Ph.D.

DARTMOUTH COLLEGE PRESS | Hanover, New Hampshire

Dartmouth College Press
An imprint of University Press of New England
www.upne.com
© 2012 Rosemarie Scolaro Moser
All rights reserved
Manufactured in the United States of America
Designed by Vicki Kuskowski
Typeset in Aldus, Din, Tasse, and Akzidenz Grotesk
by Passumpsic Publishing

University Press of New England is a member of the
Green Press Initiative. The paper used in this book meets
their minimum requirement for recycled paper.

For permission to reproduce any of the material in this book,
contact Permissions, University Press of New England,
One Court Street, Suite 250, Lebanon NH 03766;
or visit www.upne.com

Library of Congress Cataloging-in-Publication Data
Moser, Rosemarie Scolaro.
Ahead of the game: the parents' guide to youth sports concussion /
Rosemarie Scolaro Moser—1st ed.
p. cm.
Includes bibliographical references and index.
ISBN 978-1-61168-224-3 (pbk.: alk. paper)—
ISBN 978-1-61168-274-8 (ebook)
1. Pediatric sports medicine—Handbooks, manuals, etc.
2. Sports injuries in children—Handbooks, manuals, etc.
3. Brain—Concussion. I. Title.
II. Title: Parents' guide to youth sports concussion.
RC1218.C45M67 2012
617.4'81044—dc23   2011052464

5 4 3 2 1

To Serena Rose

Love your brain,
love your sport.

The information in this book is meant to provide guidance and education regarding sports concussion in youth. However, it is not meant to substitute for medical advice and evaluation by a licensed health care professional. Whenever a concussion or other injury is suspected, please immediately consult your doctor or the local emergency department. Be advised that medical research, guidelines, and treatments for concussion continue to rapidly evolve. The information presented here is current only as of the time it was written. It is important to keep abreast of changes in treatment guidelines to ensure that the most effective, up-to-date concussion care and management is provided to your child. Finally, readers should be aware that when case studies are described in this book, patients' names have been changed to protect their privacy.

Contents

Appendixes

Foreword

I have many fond memories from my days growing up in Paterson, New Jersey, including long afternoons spent on the football field, and playing third base for the baseball team at St. John the Baptist High. But back then we didn't know much about sports-related concussion, or the dangers that sometimes lurk on the athletic field.

These days, a growing body of research has indicated that concussions are much more serious than we once realized, and occur much more frequently than we ever thought possible. Each year there are as many as 3.8 million sports-related brain injuries in the United States, many of which affect children younger than eighteen. More and more studies suggest that multiple concussions may be associated with chronic brain deterioration and dementia over time. And though we are only just beginning to understand the long-term effects of sports-related concussions, the findings can no longer be ignored. As co-chair of the Congressional Brain Injury Task Force and sponsor of HR 1347, the Concussion Treatment and Care Tools Act (CONTACT), I have encouraged a nationwide commitment to protecting our student athletes.

I, along with Congressman Todd Platts of Pennsylvania, introduced the CONTACT Act, the first federal legislation designed to prevent and protect against youth concussion, after the tragic football-related death of Ryne Dougherty, a New Jersey high school student from my district. In October 2008, Dougherty died from a brain hemorrhage after making a tackle during a junior varsity game. Even though Dougherty had sustained a concussion in practice roughly three weeks earlier, he had been cleared to play by his doctor. It was only after his death, however, that we learned Dougherty had been complaining to teammates about a lingering post-concussion headache. He should not have been allowed back on the field so soon.

Tragically, this is not a lone occurrence—there are many young athletes and families who have been scarred by the devastation of traumatic brain injury. Dougherty was actually the third New Jersey teenager to die between the months of August and October 2008, after sustaining a football-related injury; his was at least the fifth football-related death of a teen in the United States that year.

Our schools and communities must be prepared to create a safe sports environment for our children, an environment where the risk of concussion is low and concussion identification and treatment is of the best quality we can possibly provide. We need to gather our finest scientists, experts, and policy makers to develop strong, research-based guidelines that address the prevention, identification, treatment, and management of concussions in all school-aged children. We need to develop reasonable, consistent standards for return to play after an injury. We need to educate young athletes and the adults who care for them, so that all are mindful and cautious in the handling of sports-related concussion. And we need to do so in a culture that continues to honor and enjoy the camaraderie and skill-building benefits of organized athletics.

We now know that the best helmets, mouth guards, and other protective equipment are not enough to prevent concussion. We now know that no child should return to the field without a thorough examination by a licensed health care practitioner who understands sports-related concussion in kids. We now know that preseason, baseline neuropsychological testing, coupled with post-concussion testing, greatly enhances our ability to determine when an athlete is ready to return to play. Despite this knowledge, most schools do not have such testing programs in place, and for schools that do, concussion policies vary from state to state. A child's brain should not be treated differently based on where he or she lives. With the implementation of the CONTACT Act, in particular the creation of federal concussion-management policies, there will be greater uniformity across our country, so that we can make school sports safe for all of our children.

I am honored to be included in this guidebook on sports concussion in student athletes, and I commend Dr. Rosemarie Moser on her efforts to educate coaches, students, and parents. I hope that you, the reader, will become inspired in your commitment and dedication to tackling this public health menace, which threatens the health and safety of our young men and women. Together, let's make sports safe for all and protect the brains and bodies of our children.

THE HONORABLE BILL PASCRELL JR.
United States House of Representatives
New Jersey Eighth Congressional District
Co-chair, Congressional Brain Injury Task Force

Acknowledgments

This book could not have been written without the kind contributions, guidance, and support of many. I wish to thank all those young athletes and families whose ideas, thoughts, and questions helped structure the tone and content of this book. I also want to thank my colleagues and staff at the Sports Concussion Center of New Jersey for their passion and commitment to the management and treatment of sports concussion. In addition, I thank my family: my parents, Nat and Mary; my husband, Bob; my children, Alex and Rachel; my son-in-law, Jim; and my new granddaughter, Serena Rose, for being companions on the journey of this book creation. In particular . . . Alex, you have taught me so much about the love of sports; you are the inspiration for this book.

Much appreciation to my special colleague and co-researcher, Phil Schatz, whose sound, cool judgment provided important editing and suggestions. Thanks to my agent, Bob DiForio, and publisher, Stephen Hull, for their strong interest and belief in this book. Especially, many thanks to Courtney Hargrave for her intelligent, creative ideas, and for her assistance in the publication of this book.

I also wish to thank the following individuals who in some way touched this book by their commitment to this important topic and their support of my work (in alphabetical order): Chris Barbrack, Lindsay Barton, Dorothy Bedford, Sheryl Berardinelli, Mary Ann Canzano, Harry Carson, the Honorable William Chatfield, Phil DeFina, Brooke de Lench, Tracy Druckenbrod, Rose Hacking, Luke Hensel, Ron Jaworksi, Robin Karpf, Rich Lisk, Monika Madan, Beth Myerowitz, U.S. Rep. Bill Pascrell Jr., Frank Webbe, and Eric Zillmer.

AHEAD OF THE GAME

INTRODUCTION

My son, Alex, has always been pretty adventurous. In high school, he started his own mountain bike racing team, taking it upon himself to recruit riders, order uniforms, and solicit sponsors. By college, he had added road cycling to his athletic repertoire. And these days, he's training to be a race car driver. But before all that, there was ice hockey.

At five and six years old, the age when Alex first started playing, ice hockey is actually pretty tame; the kids spend the majority of time racing after a wandering puck. But by age eleven or twelve, when they're suddenly allowed to *check*—basically, to use their bodies as moving barricades—well, that's when things get a little crazy. Shortly after Alex graduated to playing bantam-level defense, the family drove up to Bridgewater, New Jersey, to cheer him on in an end-of-season playoff game against a notoriously rough team—and I'm talking about *the parents*. By the time we took our seats in the bleachers, sticks were flying. Tensions were mounting. I held my breath as one player after another was sent crashing into the boards.

I was a terrible hockey mom. Every time someone fell to the ice or slammed into another player, I shot up from the stands, angled forward to see who it was, and prayed for no broken collarbones, arms, legs, or heads. It was only when the last little player had skated off the ice, trading in his helmet and pads for a cherry-red Gatorade, that I could finally relax. You might say I was overly worrisome. But it's hard not to be when you're a mom . . . *and* a neuropsychologist.

1

Back in the mid-1990s, the concept of youth sports–related concussion was almost unknown to the general public. After years spent studying the effects of mild traumatic brain injury (mTBI), however, I knew what most other parents and coaches did not: children sustain concussions at alarming rates—research shows that as many as 63 percent of high school students, for example, have already had *at least* one.[1] Contrary to popular belief, you don't have to hit your head to sustain a concussion, nor do you have to lose consciousness or "black out." Children, in particular, might not exhibit the first symptoms until *days* after a particularly hard hit or a rough tackle, which makes diagnosing a concussion at the time of injury not only difficult, but often impossible—even for a trained specialist.

By the time my son's high-stakes hockey game had ended, the opposing team had managed to slip the puck past our goalie. It was a disappointing loss—eliminated from the playoffs in the first round. As usual, Alex changed in the locker room, packed up his equipment, and met his older sister Rachel and me at the rink entrance. We walked to our car together while Rachel, then just a teenager, chattered away. So I didn't notice until we had begun the long drive home that Alex was very quiet. He didn't attack the snacks I had packed, even though he was usually voraciously hungry after a game. I asked him a few conversational questions, which he answered correctly . . . but slowly. He claimed that he was just tired, and barely spoke for the remainder of the trip.

Although he repeatedly insisted that he felt "fine," I knew that my son's demeanor just wasn't quite right. I also knew that he would do his best not to alarm *me*; Alex had grown well accustomed to having a concussion specialist for a mother, so he was used to my constant anxiety around and (sometimes overbearing) attention to the subject of his mental health. I kept an eye on him all that night, poking my head into his dark room every few hours and listening for the rhythmic sounds of his breath rising and falling, just to be safe, and by the next morning, he seemed completely back to normal. Maybe, despite my worst fears, he hadn't suffered a concussion after all? Besides, the hockey season had ended—there would be no more games for a while—so the family could rest easy now. At least for a while.

It wasn't that long ago when a rough tackle or a "bell-ringer" was something we thought athletes should be able to walk off or play through. But a sudden combination of factors—including proposed federal legislation for concussion management in schools, a series of multimillion-dollar lawsuits brought by victims of concussion, and a growing fixation on the long-term health of professional athletes—has completely changed the way we view head injuries. Seemingly overnight, the need for increased concussion awareness and management has turned into a national media frenzy.

As sports fans everywhere know, it's now practically impossible to watch a televised game without witnessing a rough tackle or a hard hit that results in a concussion, or to hear commentators provide updates on the recovery of high-profile concussed athletes.[2] Perhaps that's because in the National Football League (NFL) alone, 154 concussions were sustained in practices and games between the start of the preseason and the eighth week of the 2010 regular season, a 21 percent increase over the number of concussions sustained in 2009.[3] Those statistics, by the way, were tallied even *after* the NFL started fining players up to $100,000 for helmet-to-helmet hits and other "dangerous" tackles—even in instances where the offending play was never flagged by an official—in a hugely controversial effort to curb sports-induced concussions and ratchet up player safety.[4] Some players, coaches, agents, and fans have called the new measures "unfair" or suggested that the NFL has gone soft; James Harrison of the Pittsburgh Steelers, for example, a notoriously rough player and an outspoken critic of the initiative, tweeted that "the people making the rules at the NFL are idiots."[5] Harrison racked up four separate penalties—for a total of $125,000—between October and December 2010.[6,7]

Head injuries, of course, are not confined to the football field. Sidney Crosby, a professional hockey player for the Pittsburgh Penguins and a recipient of the Lester B. Pearson award (given to the most valuable player, or MVP, as determined by the members of the National Hockey League

[NHL] Players' Association), and considered by many to be "the next Wayne Gretzky," made national news in January 2011 after sustaining a concussion that kept him out of the remaining 2010–2011 season.[8] Crosby's hit came just one month after Derek Boogaard of the New York Rangers suffered a career-ending concussion during an on-ice fight with Matt Carkner of the Ottawa Senators; Boogaard died five months later, after ingesting a lethal combination of alcohol and prescription painkillers.[9]

In the past few years, the buzz around sports-related concussions has become so all-consuming that it now extends to the realm of virtual sports. The latest version of the wildly popular *Madden NFL* video game series, which has sold 90 million copies, is realistic enough not only to show players receiving concussions, but also to sideline those players for the remainder of the game. Gone are depictions of helmet-to-helmet hits and tackles of defenseless players. NFL commentator and Pro Football Hall of Fame coach John Madden, for whom the game is named, explained to the *New York Times* that the changes were made to *Madden 12* (released in August 2011) to educate youngsters: "It starts with young kids—they start in video games. I think the osmosis is if you get a concussion, that's a serious thing and you shouldn't play. We want that message to be strong."[6]

Concussion education and management programs—already mandatory in the NFL, NHL, and other professional sports leagues—are now gaining entry to high school and collegiate athletic programs at lightning speed. For the first time in history, you may be asked to sign a consent form acknowledging the risks and dangers of concussion before your son or daughter is allowed to participate in school-sponsored sports. If you're a resident of Washington State, signing a consent form isn't just a polite suggestion; it's a legal requirement—the "Zackery Lystedt Law," one of the most stringent youth sports concussion-prevention laws in the country, was enacted in May 2009. Thirty-four other states currently have some kind of concussion awareness program or legislation on the books (another ten or so states have legislation pending).

This overnight obsession with the prevention and management of head injuries, both in professional sports and in our schools, begs an obvious question: what's with all the urgency? The answer, it turns out, is relatively simple. A growing body of research has recently uncovered truths about concussion that scientists never before understood, and the findings have been nothing short of terrifying.

***

You could say that Dave Duerson was destined for greatness. As a high school student growing up in Muncie, Indiana, he excelled at football, basketball, and baseball. He was also a member of the National Honor Society, and an accomplished player of the sousaphone with the Musical Ambassadors All-American Band. In 1979, the year he graduated, he was invited to play professional baseball with the Los Angeles Dodgers, but instead, he chose to go to college.[10]

Duerson enrolled at the University of Notre Dame, where he became a four-year starter on the Fighting Irish football team. He became a captain and MVP during his senior season and graduated with honors in 1983. Later that same year, he married his girlfriend, Alicia. Together they went on to have four children, a daughter and three sons.

After graduation, Duerson was drafted into the NFL. His career spanned ten years, and he played in turn for the Chicago Bears, the New York Giants, and the Phoenix Cardinals. He was a four-time Pro Bowl safety and a two-time Super Bowl champion, as well as a recipient of the NFL Humanitarian of the Year award. After retiring in 1993, he went on to operate a string of successful businesses. He even earned an executive education certificate from Harvard Business School.

By the mid-2000s, however, some fifteen years after his retirement from professional football, Duerson's seemingly charmed life had begun to unravel. He was charged with battery against his wife, and their twenty-five-year marriage ended in divorce. His business fell into receivership, and he lost his home to foreclosure. Having grown increasingly angry and agitated, he eventually admitted to friends that he was battling depression. And by late 2010, Duerson was convinced that he had developed *chronic traumatic encephalopathy* (CTE), sometimes known as "gridiron dementia," a relatively new medical condition that was making waves in the sports world. As many as twenty deceased professional football players had already been found to have brain damage indicative of the disease, which includes symptoms such as headaches, insomnia, memory loss, behavioral and mood disorders, violence, and suicidal thoughts. On February 17, 2011, Duerson committed suicide by shooting himself in the abdomen, but not before writing a sad, simple note: "Please, see that my brain is given to the NFL's brain bank."[11]

The concept of concussion, of course, is not new; in fact, references to concussion and its symptoms appear in medical texts dating back to ancient Greece. Nor is the concept of dementia or neurodegenerative disease associated with *repetitive* concussions. In 1928, a doctor named Harrison Stanford Martland was the first to describe the tremors, speech problems, and confusion that plagued many professional boxers after a lifetime spent fighting in the ring (and sustaining one blow after another to the head). Martland called the condition *dementia pugilistica*, more commonly known today as boxer's dementia or punch-drunk syndrome.[12] Based partly on Martland's findings, medical professionals have been calling for a ban on professional boxing since the early 1950s. It wasn't until 2002, however, that researchers first began to realize that other athletes—most notably football players, wrestlers, and even military veterans—were showing signs of long-term, cumulative, debilitating brain damage, and that participation in sports was likely to blame.

Neuropathologist Bennet Omalu, MD, was working in the medical examiner's office in Pittsburgh when the body of "Iron Mike" Webster, a former center for the Pittsburgh Steelers and member of the Pro Football Hall of Fame, was brought in for a routine autopsy.[13] Much like Duerson's, Webster's life had deteriorated considerably since his days as a four-time Super Bowl champion; he suffered from headaches, hearing loss, depression, amnesia, and dementia. He was homeless and destitute, and spent his last few years living out of his pickup truck. Webster's official cause of death was heart failure, but Dr. Omalu—on a hunch—

wondered if the repetitive head injuries Webster had sustained over the course of his sixteen-year professional football career might have been to blame for such a tragic downward spiral. Omalu decided to search for visible evidence of brain damage and, after a special and painstaking analysis of brain tissue samples, he found it: large deposits of something called *tau*, a protein found in brain cells. Tau pathology is generally associated with Alzheimer's disease, but the magnitude of damage Omalu had discovered was unprecedented in someone so young (Webster was fifty when he died). Omalu identified the disease as chronic traumatic encephalopathy, or CTE, and published his findings in the prestigious medical journal *Neurosurgery* in 2005.[14, 15]

Since that groundbreaking discovery, more than twenty former football players, thirty former boxers, and a handful of hockey players, wrestlers, and other athletes have been found with signs of CTE in postmortem exams. Like Duerson, some of those athletes died of self-inflicted wounds after years spent suffering from depression and dementia. Andre Waters of the Philadelphia Eagles shot himself in November 2006 at age forty-four. Terry Long of the Pittsburgh Steelers died at age forty-five after drinking antifreeze. Chris Benoit, a former WWE wrestler, hanged himself in June 2007 after murdering his wife and child. In fact, the sheer rate at which new cases of CTE are being discovered (and the tragedy of so many untimely deaths) has led to the creation of the Center for the Study of Traumatic Encephalopathy, a research collaboration between Boston University Medical Center and the Sports Legacy Institute, as well as a growing library of deceased athletes' brains[16]—the "brain bank" to which Duerson referred in his suicide note. (In May 2011 it was announced that Duerson's fears had been well founded: he *did* have brain damage, particularly to the parts of the brain that control judgment, impulse, mood, and memory. Researchers believe that CTE not only caused Duerson's symptoms, but motivated his desire to end his life.)[17, 18] More than 100 living NFL players have pledged to donate their brains when they die.

Though CTE has been recognized for only a few years now, it was originally thought to be the province of retired (read: *older*) professional athletes, guys who had spent a lifetime getting pummeled on the ice, on the turf, or in the ring. (Duerson, for example, was involved in more than 550 tackles during the years he played with the Chicago Bears; and some doctors likened the hits Webster took throughout his high school, college, and professional football career to the equivalent of 25,000 automobile crashes.) But more recent research suggests that it is possible to develop CTE at much younger ages than previously thought possible. Chris Henry of the Cincinnati Bengals was only twenty-six when he died in a motor vehicle accident, but researchers found evidence of CTE in his brain, even though he had never been formally diagnosed with a concussion during his time in the NFL or during his college career at West Virginia University.[19, 20] In September 2010, the brain autopsy of twenty-one-year-old University of Pennsylvania football player Owen Thomas revealed that he, too, was in the early stages of CTE. Like Henry, Thomas was never actually diagnosed with a concussion at any point in his career, yet he hanged himself in his off-campus apartment after what friends and family described as a "sudden and uncharacteristic emotional collapse."[21] Researchers have also revealed the shocking findings of the *beginnings* of CTE in the brain of an eighteen-year-old high school football player (though this athlete, whose name has been withheld from the media, is not considered to have had full-blown CTE at the time of his death).[22]

The concerns here are obvious: CTE is a devastating disease with catastrophic effects, and it's showing up in athletes of increasingly younger ages—even in amateurs, even in high schoolers, even in kids who were never diagnosed with a concussion in the first place. Are children who sustain concussions, therefore, at greater risk for developing depression, dementia, or Alzheimer's disease later in life, just like professional athletes? And if so, then how many concussions does it take, and of what severity, before the symptoms begin to appear? Some experts are so distressed by these findings that they've wondered if kids should even be allowed to play contact or collision sports: "There is no reason, no medical justification, for any child younger than eighteen to play football, period," Omalu told the medical news service *MedPage Today*.[23] In the fall of 2011, noted concussion expert Dr. Robert Cantu, co-director of the Center for the Study of Traumatic Encephalopathy at Boston University School of Medicine, further upped the ante: "[I am] recommending that nobody under the age of fourteen be involved in collision sports."[24]

Although CTE wasn't formally identified until the mid-2000s—several years after my son had graduated beyond the youth hockey leagues of suburban New Jersey—doctors (if not parents and coaches) still knew plenty about the dangers of concussion in kids. For one thing, children are more vulnerable than adults to getting concussions, their symptoms are often more severe, their recovery typically takes longer, and they're more likely to suffer lasting effects—everything from physical problems, such as headaches and dizziness, to cognitive and intellectual problems, such as difficulty concentrating in class. Youth who've already sustained a concussion are four to six times more likely to get another.[25] They are also at risk for *second impact syndrome* (SIS), a medical event that occurs when a young athlete experiences a second head injury before fully recovering from the first. SIS causes severe and irreversible brain damage; it is fatal in up to half the individuals who suffer from it.

As a neuropsychologist, I know just how delicate a child's developing brain really is, and when Alex was playing hockey, I saw one too many youngsters sent back to the ice too soon. But as a hockey mom, I wanted my son to be an athlete and to experience the benefits of team play. Sports provide our children with a platform for setting and achieving goals, for learning discipline, and for building team skills. The athletics field is often the place where children first learn to take pride in their successes, as well as graciously accept defeat. Besides, plenty of studies show that children who play sports have stronger self-esteem and perform better in school, not to mention the health and fitness benefits associated with organized athletics.[26, 27]

So, I made it my personal mission to promote the protection and care of young brains. Starting in the mid-1990s, I began giving talks and distributing educational materials about the risk of sports-related brain injury. I created a free baseline and concussion-testing program for kids, modeled on the practices of the NHL. I collected data and published research on the effects of concussion in children. And in 2009, I opened the Sports Concussion Center of New Jersey.

I can't honestly say, however, that the response to concussion identification and management in kids has always been positive and welcoming—the information is extremely new and, frankly, frightening. Some parents don't want to acknowledge that their children's brains could be affected just by playing football, especially if those parents are former athletes themselves. (If you grew up playing sports in the 1960s, '70s, or '80s, you know that a bell-ringer was something you were supposed to shake off quickly, downplay, ignore, or outright lie about—anything to get back in the huddle.) Some coaches don't want to admit that they've returned kids to the playing field after a hit as long as their pupils looked normal and they could remember their own name. Some physicians are still skeptical about the most recent research, because they didn't learn much about youth concussion in their medical school classrooms. And I'm quite certain that my son was often embarrassed to have a frenzied concussion doctor for a mother.

But the truth is that our children are at greater risk of concussion than ever before. In a culture that worships celebrity athletes, kids are playing multiple sports starting at earlier ages, and playing those sports year-round. With the passage of Title IX in 1972, the legislation that required equal access to athletic opportunities, more girls began to participate in sports than had done so in any previous generation.[28] High school sports participation, for example, has grown from 4 million children during the 1971–1972 school year to more than 7 million in 2005–2006.[29] A growing number of children also engage in nontraditional athletic activity outside of school (often without training or guidance), such as mountain biking, rollerblading, skateboarding, snowboarding, and other sports commonly classified as "Xtreme." Perhaps not surprisingly, all of that running, jumping, kicking, and tackling puts our kids at greater risk of injury.

In the past ten years, the number of eight- to thirteen-year-olds with a sports-related concussion has doubled, while the number of fourteen-to nineteen-year-olds seeking treatment for head injuries has increased by more than 200 percent.[30] As I've already mentioned, one study found that more than half of all high school students had suffered at least one concussion; a recent Massachusetts survey revealed that 18 percent of high school students and 21 percent of middle school students had suffered a concussion *within the previous year*.[31] And approximately 500,000 children between birth and age fourteen visit the emergency room (ER) annually as a result of a mild traumatic brain injury (mTBI). That's a *lot* of concussions.

Yet those figures may actually be gross understatements; concussions often go misdiagnosed or unreported for two main reasons. First, children are often unwilling or unable to let us know when something may be wrong. Research tells us that high school students, in particular, often don't report symptoms of concussion because they don't want to leave the game or "let their teammates down."[32] And sometimes, kids just don't know any better. According to a recent study of Canadian youth, only 25–50 percent of young athletes were even able to name a single symptom.[33]

Second, the science of youth sports concussion is a highly specialized and rapidly evolving field of medicine, so an alarming number of people—including parents, coaches, athletic trainers, and most physicians—just aren't up to date on the latest research. I can't tell you how many times I've heard a parent say, "She didn't hit her head during the game, so it can't be a concussion," even though—contrary to popular opinion—you don't have to hit your head to sustain a brain injury. I cringe every time I hear, "My doctor said it wasn't a concussion because the CT scan was negative," even though CT (computerized tomography, also called CAT) scans and MRIs (magnetic resonance imaging) are typically used to identify structural brain damage such as brain swelling or brain bleeding; rarely do signs of a concussion show up on a routine neuroimaging. Not long ago, the mother of one of my teenage patients told me that the consulting neurologist had insisted that—despite continuing headache, fatigue, muscle slowness, and poor memory test results, *months* after the initial injury—her daughter's concussion wasn't "serious" because she had never lost consciousness or blacked out. Yet, we know that loss of consciousness alone does not determine the severity of a head injury.[34] In fact, severity can't be fully determined until *after* that patient has recovered. More recently, I was giving a talk at a hospital education program for physicians when a neurologist in the audience challenged the notion that mental and physical exertion has anything to do with recovery from brain injuries. He advises his high school patients to continue engaging in normal life activities, he said, even though in clinical practice mental and physical rest is the single most important aspect of concussion treatment and recovery.

I have seen too many tearful, heartbroken young athletes who will never again play a game they love because they've already sustained multiple concussions—I'm talking about ten-, eleven-, and twelve-year-olds, children who will miss out completely on the benefits of high school sports. This kind of loss, though tragic, is a frequent and common occurrence. I want to change all that.

This book is aimed at helping parents understand, prevent, identify, and seek treatment for concussion in their kids. I'll explain what to do if you think your child may have sustained a concussion, and how to find a doctor in your area who specializes in brain injuries. I'll describe how baseline or pre-concussion testing can help you make an informed decision about when to allow your child back on the field, rink, or court. I'll provide help and guidance for parents whose children play in a community sports league without concussion-testing programs or athletic trainers in place. And I'll explain how proposed state and federal legislation may affect you and your children.

It is my sincere hope that parents, coaches, nurses, athletic trainers, teachers, and doctors will embrace the information, and will use it to prolong the athletic careers of our kids. It is my hope that "brain hygiene" will become part of standard preventive care. Our children undergo routine physical exams and regular dental checkups. Shouldn't we also be working to protect their most vital organ of all—the brain?

Test Your Concussion Knowledge

Is each of the following statements *true* or *false*? You'll find the correct answers, along with an explanation of each, in Appendix B at the end of the book.

1. *True or false?* A concussion generally isn't considered severe unless the athlete lost consciousness or "blacked out."

2. *True or false?* Properly fitting helmets and mouth guards prevent concussion in children.

3. *True or false?* Adolescent boys are more likely than adolescent girls to sustain concussions.

4. *True or false?* A sideline assessment test, in which a coach or athletic trainer asks the injured athlete a series of questions immediately following an injury, can help determine the severity of a concussion.

5. *True or false?* If a child no longer has any symptoms twenty-four hours after sustaining a mild concussion, it's safe for him or her to return to play.

6. *True or false?* The best way to diagnose a concussion is with a CT scan or MRI.

7. *True or false?* Most emergency room physicians are well trained in the management and treatment of sports concussions.

8. *True or false?* It's possible for children to experience headaches and difficulty concentrating in class for weeks after a hard hit or a rough tackle.

9. *True or false?* The "three strikes and you're out" rule, suggesting that children who have sustained three concussions should no longer be allowed to participate in school-sponsored athletics, is the result of extensive concussion management and recovery research.

10. *True or false?* There are cases where kids who are diagnosed with attention deficit hyperactivity disorder (ADHD) or other learning disabilities could actually be suffering from undiagnosed post-concussion syndrome.

1

READY, SET, LEARN!
Understanding the Young Brain

The human brain is a fascinatingly complex organ. In fact, it's arguably the most important organ in the entire body. It's the "master engineer," the planner, organizer, and conductor of all bodily functions. The brain determines how we think and feel, signals an empty stomach to growl, and guides the rhythm of the heart. When our brains are allowed to mature and grow free of injury, we are able to gain skills, enhance our mental and physical abilities, and improve the quality of our lives. But when the brain is injured or disrupted, then quirky, unexpected, and sometimes subtle changes can occur that can affect our daily functioning.

Understanding the brain is a challenging task, for one basic reason: it's just not easily accessible for research purposes. Invasive procedures are incredibly risky, and brain surgery is one of the least common of all surgical procedures. Because scientists and doctors have had less opportunity to see, feel, touch, and examine the living brain than other organs in the body, we must rely on alternative, less invasive measures to study the inner workings of the mind. Researchers have made some great strides with the use of magnetic resonance imaging (MRI) and electroencephalography (EEG), which provide us with information about the electrical activity of the brain, blood flow, and the "mapping" of different areas of brain function. Additionally, neuroscientists, specifically neuropsychologists (my area of expertise), can gather information by testing human subjects on a variety of tasks that document thinking, behavior, and emotion. These types of tasks may measure memory; attention; concentration; speed of processing; logical thinking; and speech, language, sensory, motor, and other skills.

In the most basic terms, the human brain has evolved from a "lower brain"—which triggers basic emotions, automatic behavioral responses, and motor functions—to a "higher brain," or cerebral cortex, the part of the brain that's typically gray (hence the term *gray matter*) and full of wrinkly folds. The cerebral cortex is what allows us to reason in abstract ways, to understand abstract concepts such as the past and the future, and to communicate through language. In short, it's what distinguishes us from other animals. While the lower or more primitive brain continues to function in humans, our *actions* are governed by critical oversight and reasoning from the higher brain. For example, if the lower brain triggers intense anger when, say, we get fired from our job, the cerebral cortex helps us control the impulse to scream, kick, or punch—all actions that would undoubtedly have additional negative consequences. In contrast, if a house cat (which has a less developed, more primitive cerebral cortex) feels threat or impending harm, an aggressive response—like biting or scratching—is natural and automatic, as all cat lovers know. All of that advanced cognitive activity in the human brain takes a lot of energy. In fact, the human brain uses up approximately 20–25 percent of the "energy budget" of the entire body. The brains of more primitive animals, on the other hand, require much less energy to function.

WHAT HAPPENS WHEN THE BRAIN IS INJURED?

Generally speaking, the skull acts as a sort of natural helmet for the brain, protecting it from injury. Inside the skull, the brain floats around in a cushion of *cerebrospinal fluid*, which functions as a kind of shock absorber.

Let's think back to Physics 101 for a moment. Remember Newton's first law—an object in motion stays in motion? When an individual receives a blow to the head or a strong force to the body that causes a whiplash motion, it's possible for the brain to continue traveling throughout

> ## What Happens When Things Go Wrong?
>
> The brain is composed of approximately 50 billion to 100 billion brain cells, or *neurons*, which are connected by a delicate, intricate network of fibers called *axons*. You can think about it like this: just as a power cord transfers electricity from a wall outlet to a light bulb, axons transfer electrical impulses from the brain to other parts of the body. (So, if you grabbed a hot skillet without an oven mitt, your neurons would scream, "Hey, hot pan!" and the axons would deliver the message—through your nervous system—down to your burning hand.) When the brain is healthy and functioning properly, these electrical impulses are transmitted loud and clear. But when the brain is shaken within the skull, the network of axons is stretched and sheared, affecting the axons' ability to communicate. The immediate signs of concussion, including disorientation, confusion, and dizziness, as well as the prolonged symptoms, such as headache, fatigue, and poor concentration, are the results of that injury. It's like using an old, frayed electrical cord—plug it in and your light bulb will flicker.

the cerebrospinal fluid for an instant, before slamming into the bony structures inside the skull. That impact results in a brief period of neurological impairment (confusion and amnesia are hallmark symptoms of concussion), as well as a temporary disruption of the brain's delicate electrochemical balance, triggering a cascade of chemical reactions.[1] Simply put, the brain "freaks out":

· First, calcium ions, which normally sit just outside each individual neuron (brain cell), begin to leak *into* the neurons while potassium ions leak *out*. This electrochemical shift can trigger a slowdown of cerebral blood flow, as well as an energy depletion—basically, the brain cells become too sluggish to function properly.

· As a result, the brain jumps into emergency mode. To make up for the energy depletion, it rallies all of its glucose (sugar), the body's primary source of fuel. Using up all those glucose reserves to heal the injury, however, means that other important brain processes (which need energy to run) start to slow down.

Ultimately, this chemical cascade leaves the brain in an energy crisis, which may escalate in severity over the next twenty-four to seventy-two hours as the brain attempts to heal itself.[1] This may explain why some athletes don't exhibit symptoms of a concussion (such as headaches and difficulty concentrating) until days after a hard check or a rough tackle sends them reeling. Throughout the recovery process—which can last from several days to several weeks or even longer, depending on the severity of the injury—the brain will remain in a state of metabolic depression. In other words, a concussion is *exhausting*. Mental and physical rest is critical during this time, when the brain is more vulnerable to a second injury. If the brain is shaken, hit, or overexerted again, then recovery may be prolonged, or more permanent damage may occur. My motto? Don't stress a brain when it's down.

THE VULNERABLE YOUNG BRAIN

So, we know that the brain is an amazing organ, and we know that a concussion can cause some serious damage. But here's the thing: a child's brain is more dynamic than yours or mine—it's constantly growing, changing, and building new structures. In fact, the brain doesn't reach maturity until approximately the mid-twenties, and higher cognitive functions are the last to develop. For example, the capacity for logic and abstract reasoning in a four-year-old is very different from that of a ten-year-old or twenty-one-year-old. A small child just isn't capable of solving algebraic equations, because her brain hasn't yet reached that level of development.

In the 1920s, a well-known Swiss psychologist, Jean Piaget, set out to illustrate this point by studying the developmental stages of reasoning

—from concrete to abstract—in his own children. In a classic experiment, he showed a child two identical containers, each bearing the same amount of liquid. The child acknowledged that the amount of liquid in each container was equal. Then Piaget poured the liquid from one container into a short, wide vessel, and the liquid of the second container into a tall, thin vessel. Here's what he discovered: children over the age of seven know that even though the containers may look different, the amount of liquid remains constant. Younger children, however, will insist that the tall, thin glass now holds more water. The more mature brain understands the concept of *constancy* (that is, when things remain the same under different conditions), and can coordinate different types of information from the environment, such as the amount of liquid and the change in container size, to make a more accurate judgment.[2]

Because the young brain is constantly growing and changing, we once believed—incorrectly, it turns out—that children could bounce back more quickly and heal faster. We thought they might be able to "grow out" of their injuries, whereas an adult, whose brain is more static, might be stuck with an injury. More recently, though, we've discovered that an adult is often able to use other areas of his mature, developed brain to compensate for functions in the damaged or injured area. Recovery in a young person is more elusive. When a child is injured, the young brain is forced to continue growing and maturing with that injury, and it's almost impossible to determine the myriad ways the brain may be affected over the long term. For example, if a child sustains an injury prior to reaching more abstract stages of thinking, we won't know how or if her *capacity* for abstract thinking will be affected until she reaches that particular developmental stage. In other words, the injury will affect the foundational organization of the brain over time.

Further complicating matters, the areas of the brain often affected by a concussion are the front and back regions. And the *prefrontal cortex*, for example, which handles problem solving, reasoning, and social cognition (such as the ability to make moral judgments), is located, as you might imagine, *in the front*. Now imagine your Pop Warner lineman

Did You Know . . . ?

Girls are more prone than boys to mild traumatic brain injury (mTBI). Among soccer players, girls are 68 percent more likely to sustain a concussion. Among basketball players, the odds are three to one.[4]

running his head into another player's chest, and you can see how this might be an issue.

In terms of recovery from concussions, recent research tells us that the young brain responds and adapts very differently than does the adult brain. Clinicians have observed that when compared to adults, children seem to exhibit a more pronounced delay in the onset of symptoms, so the severity of the concussion—even the diagnosis itself—might not be fully apparent until days after contact. There's even some evidence to suggest that the younger a child is, the more delayed his or her symptoms may be, and the longer it may take to recover from those symptoms. In a 2003 study, for example, high school students aged fourteen to eighteen had longer periods of "memory dysfunction" following a concussion, compared to college students aged nineteen to twenty-five.[3] *This* is why sending a child back onto the playing field too early, before he has first completed a solid course of rest, is so potentially dangerous. Children's recovery curves may also differ from those of adults—children are more likely to feel better initially, only to worsen days later. Youth also tend to experience more severe symptoms than do adults, further challenging that old notion that kids can bounce back fast.

HIS BRAIN, HER BRAIN— GENDER DIFFERENCES AND CONCUSSION

For years, scientists have been trying to pinpoint differences between male and female brains, and have struggled to interpret their findings. (For example, are boys naturally better at math? Do women have a

greater facility for language?) Here's what we *do* know: there is mounting evidence that females are more susceptible to concussion, and when
compared to males, females may often experience more severe and long-
lasting symptoms. Among soccer players, for example, girls are 68 percent more likely than boys to sustain a concussion. Among basketball
players, the odds are three to one. Females also tend to perform more
poorly than males on post-concussion testing.[5] The research begs a simple question: why? Here are the most common theories:

· Female brains are anatomically different than male brains.
For starters, male brains are typically larger than female
brains—the average adult male brain, for example, weighs
roughly 12 percent more than an adult female brain. (Of
course, size isn't a measure of intelligence, as any woman
will surely tell you.) Research also shows that women have
a thicker *corpus callosum*—the area of the brain connecting
the right and left hemispheres—which suggests that women
may be able to transfer and coordinate information from different areas of the brain more efficiently than men. (Perhaps
this is scientific evidence to support the notion of female in-
tuition?) Women also tend to have more cellular connections,
while men may have more actual neurons, or cells. Scientists
don't yet fully understand all the differences between male
and female brains, but it stands to reason that various ana-
tomical differences would account for differences in the ways
that male and female brains react and respond to injury.

· Female brains are affected by fluctuating hormones. The primary male and female sex hormones, testosterone and estrogen, account for all kinds of biological, physiological, and
emotional differences between the sexes. So perhaps it's not
surprising that differences in sex hormones may also account
for differences in the ways that boys and girls both sustain
and recover from sports-related injuries. In fact, hormones

may be the reason that girls suffer from greater and more severe injuries than do boys in general. For example, higher levels of estrogen account for greater flexibility in girls, but also "looser" joints, which may be why girls are up to ten times more likely to tear their anterior cruciate ligament or ACL, a major ligament in the knee, according to a study cited by the *New York Times*.[6] Research has indicated that girls are also more likely to develop chronic knee, hip, and back pain; shin splints; and ankle problems, among many other injuries.[6]

The brain, of course, is not immune to hormonal shifts. Some studies of epileptic women, for example, have shown that rising and falling levels of estrogen and progesterone, having to do with monthly menstruation, may make the brain more vulnerable to seizures.[7] Other studies, however, have suggested that estrogen may actually help *prevent* more serious and long-lasting brain damage after a concussion, like the kind found in cases of second impact syndrome (more on that in the next section).[8] Ultimately, how and why—and even *if*—hormonal shifts may make women and girls more susceptible to concussion we don't yet know; much more research is needed on the subject. (It's interesting to note, though, that a hormonal link to concussions would probably *not* account for a disparity of injury rates between the sexes in pre-puberty children.)

· Males typically have stronger neck muscles than do females. When someone experiences a blow to the head or torso (for example, during a football tackle), the neck muscles act as a kind of shock absorber, diffusing and displacing some of the energy from the hit. One of the reasons that children are at greater risk than adults for concussion may be that they have proportionately bigger heads, but weaker necks. Because girls also tend to have weaker neck muscles, it's speculated

that they may be less able than boys to ward off a concussive blow.

· Females *may* be more likely to acknowledge symptoms of a
concussion. Some experts believe that sociocultural differences account for higher rates of concussion among young
girls. In a society that often encourages males to toughen
up and play through the pain, for example, boys may be less
likely to admit to headaches and dizziness for fear of appear-
ing weak, or losing their spot on a lineup. But it's my opinion
that this is a dangerous theory. It's just not safe to *assume*
that a girl will let you know that she's feeling poorly just because she's a girl. As any parent of a talented female athlete
knows, girls these days are just as competitive as boys.

It's important to point out that none of these theories has actually
been proven—we're still learning exactly what causes girls to experience
concussion at higher rates than boys. It's true, though, that young girls
may be less aware of the signs and symptoms of concussion, and they
may receive less training in prevention, awareness, and management, because for so long concussions were thought to be a "boy thing." Parents
of female athletes should be just as concerned for their daughters' safety
as their sons'—or, based on these new theories, perhaps even more so.

THE DANGERS OF SECOND IMPACT SYNDROME

In addition to experiencing a delay in the onset of symptoms and an increased severity of concussion, young athletes (up to their early twen-
ties) are also at greater risk of developing a devastating condition known
as second impact syndrome, or SIS, which occurs when a child receives a
second hit before fully recovering from the first concussion. This second
injury to an already overtaxed brain can result in immediate swelling, severe neurological damage, and death, even if the second hit is a mild one.
SIS is fatal in up to one-half of the individuals who develop it.

Second Impact Syndrome: Who Is Most at Risk?

Although anyone who participates in contact or collision sports (such as football, soccer, hockey, lacrosse, basketball, or rugby) is at risk for concussion, SIS disproportionately affects youth, is most identified in American football players, and is almost always seen in adolescent or young boys, not girls. In fact, there hasn't yet been a documented case of SIS in a female. (Whether boys have some increased vulnerability to SIS in particular, because they participate in high-contact sports in greater numbers than girls, or whether SIS simply hasn't been reported in girls, we don't know.) These findings are particularly strange because, as we've already discussed, when compared to young men, young women are more susceptible to run-of-the-mill concussions. Despite the statistics, it's never safe to assume that one child is any more or less vulnerable than another to SIS. Children should *always* be removed from play after a concussion, even if the diagnosis is unclear. Better to be safe than sorry.

We don't exactly know why children are more vulnerable than adults to SIS. We do know, however, that children tend to be unaware of the symptoms of concussion in the first place, making diagnosis of the initial injury that much more difficult. (If a child doesn't understand the extent of his injury, he may be more likely to head back into the game, often without informing a parent or coach that he's been hurt or doesn't feel well.)

Such was the case for Zackery Lystedt, a thirteen-year-old football player at Tahoma Junior High in Maple Valley, Washington, who took an unusually hard hit during an afternoon game in the fall of 2006. But he decided to "shake it off" and returned to play without telling his coach about the injury. When he was hit again in the second half of the game, Lystedt developed a (then undetectable) brain hemorrhage. By the time he was rushed to the hospital, after collapsing on the field, doctors were barely able to save him. He was reportedly in and out of a coma for several months. Today, Lystedt copes with a severe disability, and will most likely need assistance for the rest of his life.[9]

In the past, there's been some controversy surrounding the legitimacy of SIS, in part due to its infrequency—between 1984 and 1991, there were only four documented cases.[10] In fact, some experts believe that the catastrophic swelling isn't caused by a second hit at all, but is actually caused by excess fluid buildup in the brain (called *cerebral edema*), and is merely a (rare) complication of the first concussion. Despite the controversy, though, SIS *is* recognized by physicians and is now being diagnosed with greater frequency, in part because more and more doctors are being taught to recognize it.

COLLISION VERSUS CONTACT SPORTS, AND THE RISK OF CONCUSSION

You may have noticed that many of the studies I've cited so far have to do with American football players. There's a simple explanation for that: American football, statistically speaking, is the most high-risk sport when it comes to concussions and long-term brain damage. Football accounts for more than half of all sports-related concussions in kids; it's estimated that 20 percent of high school football players sustain a concussion each year.[11] One reason for that involves the distinction between "contact" and "collision" sports.

There is sometimes controversy when it comes to determining the differences between contact and collision sports (some people think that rugby, for example, is not nearly as dangerous as football). But generally speaking, a collision sport is one in which the athletes hit or collide with each other—often with great force—*on purpose*. The job of an offensive lineman, for example, is to block, bring down, or otherwise impede the opposing player in order to protect the quarterback; and ice hockey players routinely check each other into the boards. A contact sport, on the other hand, is one in which the athletes may touch or make contact with one another, but with considerably less force. In basketball, for example, players may brush up against each other, but they're not supposed to tackle each other to the court. (Yet as any fan of the National Basketball Association [NBA] surely knows, players routinely slip, fall, trip, or "accidentally" collide with each other all the time.) Obviously, collision sports—including football, ice hockey, and men's lacrosse, as defined by the National Collegiate Athletic Association (NCAA)—*tend* to carry the most risk of brain injury (or any injury). These are followed by contact sports (for example, basketball and soccer), limited-contact sports (baseball, softball, and volleyball), and no-contact sports (tennis, swimming, golf, and rowing).

Another reason that football, in particular, can be so potentially dangerous has to do with the sheer force with which players make contact. Data from the NFL revealed that in open-field collisions resulting in concussion, the "striking" player was traveling approximately twenty miles per hour, and the heads of the "struck" athletes absorbed enough of that energy to travel fifteen miles per hour *after the blow*.[12] Researchers also measure the ferocity and strength of these hits and tackles in *g-forces*. Scientifically speaking, a g-force is a unit of gravity and acceleration exerted upon an object. In more general terms, g-forces are the way we measure the acceleration of an object relative to free fall. For example, zero gravity or 0 g is used to define the gravity-free conditions in outer space, when astronauts float around weightlessly inside a shuttle. Upon landing, however, astronauts may be exposed to around 3 g of force for a period of fifteen minutes or more. This is why they wear g-suits; exposure to high levels of g-force for long periods of time can lead to loss of consciousness and even death. High-speed roller coasters, on the other hand, might expose the rider to as much as 6 g, if only for a few seconds at a time. When it comes to football collisions, the *average* g-force imposed on a player is somewhere around 23 g, but the numbers often register much, much higher than that. As reported by *Time* magazine, a study of college football players by athletic trainer and researcher Dr. Kevin Guskiewicz of the University of North Carolina found that higher-end collisions range anywhere from 80–100 g; the hardest hit Guskiewicz recorded was 180 g.[13] So, how many g does it take to potentially sustain a concussion? Only about 60 or 70 g in an adult, and no word yet on g-forces in children.

Yet another concern is an athlete's exposure to what we call *subconcussive* blows. These are blows that do affect the brain (over the long term) but aren't severe enough to cause any instant symptoms. Guskiewicz has estimated that the average college football player may sustain as many as 950 to 1,100 subconcussive hits per season. "That's what we call a dose response," he told *Time* magazine in 2011. "After a certain number of hits, the damage starts to show."[13] The real danger of subconcussive blows is that, in the absence of any symptoms, players are much more likely to stay on the field. (We'll talk more about how to monitor and guard against the possible effects of subconcussive blows in Chapter 3.)

Of course, football isn't the only risky sport when it comes to brain injuries, nor is this book in any way an indictment of collision sports such as football or ice hockey. On the contrary, I'm not only a fan of these sports, I'm the official neuropsychologist for two Arena Football League (AFL) teams—the Philadelphia Soul and Trenton Steel—as well as the official neuropsychologist for the Trenton Titans professional hockey team. The reality is that *all* collision and contact sports, and even some limited-contact sports, put our kids at risk of concussion. For example, 20 percent of high school football players may sustain concussions each season, but research shows that baseball and softball players aren't far behind—19 percent of them sustain concussions, followed by 17 percent of wrestlers and 11 percent of ice hockey athletes.[14] What's more, studies estimate that one-third of all concussions in children are sustained during non-team sports such as bicycling or skateboarding.[13] In younger children, the majority of head injuries aren't associated with organized sports at all; they're most often the result of falls, or they are sustained during "free play" or recess.[15] What this means is that no child is completely exempt from the risk of concussion, and all parents need to be aware of the signs and symptoms.

THE APOE GENE—A GENETIC PREDISPOSITION TO CONCUSSION?

Is the child of athletically gifted parents more likely to become an athlete herself? Could genetics be the reason that some people excel at marathon running while others are better sprinters? Are professional athletes and Olympic champions genetically predestined for greatness? These are just a few of the questions that scientists have sought to answer since the launch of the Human Genome Project in 1989, an international research initiative aimed at mapping human DNA, as well as locating and understanding the genes that code for traits such as eye color, height, congenital disease, or athletic ability. Although the science of the genome is still a relatively new and rapidly evolving field of medicine, researchers have already been able to make some incredible discoveries about the human genome. For example, you may be familiar with BRCA (breast cancer) testing, which can uncover mutations of BRCA1 and BRCA2, the genes associated with an increased risk of developing breast cancer. It's also possible to order prenatal genetic testing to spot chromosomal disorders such as Down syndrome. Scientists have even discovered a gene that's associated with Alzheimer's disease: it's called ApoE.

Everyone inherits two copies of the ApoE gene, one from each parent, of which there are three possible variants: ApoE2, ApoE3, and ApoE4. People with one copy of ApoE4—roughly 25 percent of the general population—are around three to four times more likely to develop Alzheimer's disease than are people with ApoE2 or ApoE3. Folks with two copies have a risk factor eight to ten times as great. More recent research, however, suggests that ApoE may play a role not just in Alzheimer's, but also in the brain's ability to recover from trauma and injury, including concussion.[16]

Several studies have shown that people with ApoE4 may be more susceptible to getting concussions, may have a harder time recovering from concussions, and may be more likely to develop chronic traumatic encephalopathy (CTE), the debilitating brain damage that's been linked to repetitive concussive and subconcussive blows.[17] Remember Dr. Bennet Omalu, first mentioned in the introduction, the neuropathologist who discovered evidence of CTE in the brain of "Iron Mike" Webster? It turns out that of all the former athletes studied by Omalu's Brain Injury Research Institute, 70 percent of those with CTE also had at least one copy of ApoE4, including former WWE wrestler Chris Benoit and former Cincinnati Bengals wide receiver Chris Henry.[18] And at the Center for the Study of Traumatic Encephalopathy, researchers found ApoE4 in five out of nine athletes who also had CTE (that's 56 percent).[16] The implications are that genetics may play a larger role than concussions alone in determining who winds up with long-term degenerative brain damage or dementia.

You may be wondering: if it's possible to test for BRCA1 or Down syndrome, can you also test for the presence of ApoE4? The answer is yes. In fact, some university athletic programs, notably the Duke University football team, have considered submitting their players' DNA for genetic testing. And some private companies have started offering at-home DNA tests for parents—at a couple hundred bucks a pop—to screen for genes such as ApoE4, as well as ACTN3, sometimes colloquially referred to as the "speed gene," which *may* predispose a person to enhanced athletic ability.[16, 19]

At first blush, this might sound like a great idea. After all, if you discover your child has ApoE4, you may be more inclined to closely monitor his concussions, to insist on a longer recovery period after a concussion, or to steer him clear of riskier sports, such as football, altogether. Yet many bioethicists are strongly opposed to the use of at-home genetic tests by the general public, at least for the time being. Here's why:

· Though the research regarding the link between ApoE4 and a person's susceptibility to concussion, as well as his or her susceptibility to developing long-term brain damage, is *compelling*, it is far from concrete. In fact, some concussion experts have asserted that something called an ApoE *promoter*

> ### Did You Know . . . ?
>
> There are three different classifications of brain injury: mild, moderate, and severe. Concussions are considered mild brain injuries because there is no skull fracture, there is no intracranial bleeding or hemorrhaging, and recovery is expected. But that doesn't mean that concussions are not *serious*. After all, you'd take even a "mild" heart attack seriously, wouldn't you? The same principle applies to concussions.

may be associated with susceptibility to and recovery from brain injury, rather than the ApoE gene itself.[20] Therefore, we are still a long way from understanding the many ways that ApoE4 may or may not affect recovery from brain injuries, and at this stage, it's more likely that test results could be misunderstood or misused.

· Athletes *without* ApoE4 might feel a false sense of security about their risk of head injury, even though we know that concussions and lingering post-concussion symptoms are still common in people who don't have the gene variant. (ApoE4 is not a guarantee that you'll develop concussion complications or Alzheimer's disease; it's simply a contributing factor.)

· Although it is technically illegal for employers and insurance companies to discriminate on the basis of genetic predisposition to disease or disability—thanks to the Genetic Information Nondiscrimination Act of 2008—some experts still worry about the possibility of discrimination or the potential misuse of genetic information. (The us Food and Drug Administration [FDA] has even stepped in, prohibiting the sale of some tests and demanding a validation of the sale of others.)

· And, of course, there is the fact that some people may just not want to know that they have an increased risk for developing Alzheimer's, a devastating degenerative disease, later in life.

WHAT MULTIPLE CONCUSSIONS COULD MEAN FOR YOUR CHILD'S FUTURE

We already know that once an athlete sustains one concussion, he or she is between four and six times more likely to suffer another. A growing body of research now also suggests that the severity of concussions (and their symptoms) may worsen with each subsequent injury, regardless of how far apart the injuries occur. In other words, the damage from repeated concussions may be cumulative, compounding over time. In a study of 223 healthy high school athletes, for example, my colleagues and I discovered that athletes with a history of no or one concussion performed significantly better on tests of attention and concentration than did athletes with a history of two or more concussions.[21] In a later study, we also discovered that high school athletes with a history of two or more concussions reported more cognitive, emotional, physical, and sleep symptoms than did athletes who have experienced one or no concussions.[22] What this means is that children who have experienced more than one concussion *may* be more likely to struggle in class (sometimes failing to maintain their usual grade point average), and to have lingering physical problems such as headache, dizziness, and blurred vision. The question is, do youth who experience these subtle effects early in life become the adults who eventually exhibit symptoms of brain dysfunction, dementia, depression, and other emotional disorders? Could these subtle changes in memory and concentration be a precursor of things to come?

As I outlined in my introduction, there's been a growing focus in the media lately regarding the alarming behavioral changes in some retired professional athletes, based largely on the recent findings of CTE. The NFL, in particular, has come under increasingly intense scrutiny based on its reluctance to acknowledge the dangers and long-term consequences of repetitive brain injury. So much so, in fact, that a series of congressional hearings was launched in 2009 to investigate the latest brain injury research and to discuss possible compensation for injured professional athletes. This exposure has finally prompted the NFL to institute some new concussion-management policies, including fining players for hits and tackles that are deemed "dangerous" and hanging a poster, detailing the risks of concussions, in team locker rooms across the country. That kind of commitment to concussion awareness, however, isn't necessarily a view shared by everyone. Hall of Fame quarterback Troy Aikman, who retired in early 2001 after a twelve-year career and as many as ten concussions, has chosen not to comment on concussions—neither his own nor other players'—in part because he doesn't want people to think that he's suffering from any post-concussion symptoms: "I don't want to be looked at as one who is experiencing some of these things that other players talk about," he told the *Milwaukee Journal-Sentinel* in January 2011. "Because I'm not."[23]

Parents may have a difficult time admitting that multiple concussions may put their children at risk for long-term effects or may even necessitate a removal from the sport they love. But unfortunately, we just don't know how many concussions it takes before a few "bell-ringers" turn into irreversible brain damage. What's clear is the need to protect young brains from injury and, when an injury does occur, the importance of giving children adequate time to heal.

Chapter 1 Review

· We still know very little about concussions from a scientific, research-based perspective.

· Because young brains are more vulnerable than adult brains, we should avoid applying the same treatment and management principles to athletes of all ages. Kids often experience worse symptoms than do adults, often take longer to recover, and are at greater risk for second impact syndrome, or SIS.

· Don't neglect female athletes. Girls are more susceptible than boys to concussion.

· The effects of concussion are subtle, yet enduring. Children who sustain multiple concussions—even spaced years apart —may be more prone to experience problems with attention, concentration, and cognitive development.

2

IS IT REALLY A CONCUSSION?

Identifying a leg injury is usually pretty simple, especially when a child limps off the field after a tackle or clutches his knee in pain. But identifying a brain injury is considerably more complex. Unless the athlete exhibits very obvious signs (such as blacking out, having difficulty keeping his balance, or having difficulty remembering his own name), chances are he'll walk off the field or skate off the ice, and no one will be the wiser. Even when a brain injury *is* suspected by a coach or athletic trainer, old-school methods of sideline testing—the "how many fingers am I holding up?" routine—just aren't effective. So how are you supposed to know if your child has really sustained a concussion?

WHAT IS A CONCUSSION?

The word *concussion* comes from the Latin terms *concutere* (shaking) or *concussus* (striking together), but numerous official definitions have been scrutinized and refined over the years. That's largely because our understanding of the causes and effects of concussion has changed considerably over time. Whereas, say, a fractured tibia has a clear, precise definition—the leg bone is fractured or broken—a concussion is harder to diagnose. Medical organizations such as the American Academy of Neurology and the National Athletic Trainer's Association, as well as various researchers and medical experts, are constantly revising their official positions on identifying and treating brain injuries.

What's generally agreed upon is that a concussion is what we call a *diffuse* injury, meaning that it is widespread in the brain, affecting many parts (as opposed to a *focal* injury, which affects just one specific part of the brain; a hemorrhage, for example, is a type of focal injury). In other words, a concussion isn't a wound you can see, like a bleeding cut or a broken leg. Rather, a concussion is the period of *neurological impairment* that occurs as a result of a hit, tackle, fall, or impact. It doesn't matter how brief or how extended that impairment is, or how seemingly mild or severe it is at the time of injury—it's still a concussion. And in fact, a concussion that seems severe, like the kind that results in a loss of consciousness, may actually wind up being a lesser injury than one that doesn't initially produce any symptoms. As I've mentioned before, it's possible for an athlete to feel better for a while, only to worsen a few days later.

How a concussion occurs is pretty straightforward—the individual receives either a blow to the head or a strong force to the body, such as a whiplash motion, which causes the brain to shake within the skull. Scientifically speaking, there are two mechanisms for a sports-related concussive injury: (1) *acceleration-deceleration* and (2) *rotational*. Acceleration-deceleration occurs when the head is jolted in a straight line, either forward or back, and then stops suddenly. Rotational injury occurs when the head rotates or twists in reaction to a blow. For example, when a boxer takes a right hook to the jaw, his head may whip around to the side. Or, if a football player sustains a tackle from his blind side, his head may turn sharply as he goes down. Researchers suspect that rotational hits, which twist the lower base of the brain at its interface with the spinal cord, cause more severe symptoms; so it's the *force*, not necessarily a blow to the head specifically, that results in injury. (Technically speaking, there is a third mechanism for a concussive injury: military personnel are sometimes concussed when subjected to the detonation of a roadside bomb, improvised explosive device (IED), or other explosion. Though these "blast injuries" are different from acceleration-deceleration and rotational impacts, they often produce similar signs and symptoms.)

34

Did You Know . . . ?

A growing number of cell phone apps are available to help identify concussions. For example, the ImPACT concussion awareness tool (ImCAT) provides summaries of common symptoms, presented as a series of check boxes and pull-down screens. Although these types of tools might be helpful from an educational perspective (by helping kids learn the signs and symptoms of brain injury), and may aid in documenting immediate signs so the information can be given to a doctor, it's important to remember that concussions are serious—you can't rely on your smartphone for health care diagnosis or treatment. If you suspect that your child has sustained a concussion, seek advice from a medical professional.

RECOGNIZING THE SIGNS AND SYMPTOMS: WHY SIDELINE TESTING ISN'T A DIAGNOSTIC TOOL

When an athlete experiences a hard hit or a rough tackle, trips, or falls to the ground, a variety of immediate signs may be present. Confusion, disorientation, feeling dazed or "foggy," visual disturbance or blurred vision, dizziness, balance problems, amnesia, nausea or vomiting, loss of consciousness, headache, numbness or tingling, fatigue, changes in emotional status or behavior, and other changes in sensory, motor, or nervous system functioning are all hallmarks of a brain injury. It takes only *one* of these symptoms, however, to suspect a concussion. If any of these signs are present, the athlete should be immediately removed from play and examined by a licensed health care professional who has been trained specifically in concussion diagnosis and treatment.

On the sideline, it's usually a coach, athletic trainer, or sometimes even an attentive parent whose job it is to check for these signs. Certified athletic trainers, in particular, have generally been trained in concussion identification and will often consult routine questionnaires or checklists. The Standardized Assessment of Concussion (SAC), for example, features questions that look at memory, attention, concentration, and orientation[1]—so your child may be asked simple orientation questions (what day of the week is it?), concentration questions (list the months of the year in reverse order), and memory questions (listen to a random list of words, and then recite those words in order). All of these questions are used to determine how oriented and aware the athlete is at the time of injury, and are scored on a scale from 1 to 30.

What's useful about tools like the SAC is that they can help to *document* the signs and severity of symptoms at the time of injury; that information can then be forwarded to a physician or neuropsychologist to aid in monitoring the treatment and recovery of the athlete. But checklists and questionnaires alone are not *diagnostic*, meaning that they cannot be used by a layperson to diagnose a concussion, nor can they be used to determine the severity of a concussion. It doesn't matter how well your child "scores" on a sideline assessment test; even if he scores a "perfect" 30, he should not be allowed back on the field—not even if it's the championship game, the home team is down by three, and there are two minutes left in the fourth quarter. The mere presence of any symptom, for any length of time, may indicate a brain injury. The sideline test is merely a tool.

Because each brain injury is unique and must be evaluated and treated on an individual basis, it's nearly impossible to develop an effective universal grading system to determine the severity of a concussion. Of course, that hasn't stopped experts from trying; more than twenty published grading systems may still be in use by coaches and trainers across the country.[2] But it's important to understand that none of these systems is research based, and all of them are arbitrary. For example, in 1997 the American Academy of Neurology proposed the following grading system to classify the severity of a concussion (based almost entirely on whether the athlete had lost consciousness):[3] grade 1, a "mild" concussion, would be your seemingly run-of-the-mill event; the athlete might feel confused or "dinged," but did not lose consciousness or black out, and symptoms resolved in less than fifteen minutes. After a grade 2, or "moderate" concussion, an athlete's symptoms might persist for

What to Watch For: Initial Signs and Symptoms of Concussion

· confusion

· disorientation

· dazed or "foggy" feeling

· amnesia

· loss of consciousness

· visual disturbances (blurred vision or sensitivity to light)

· tinnitus (ringing in the ears) and sound sensitivity

· dizziness

· balance problems

· nausea or vomiting

· headache

· numbness or tingling

· fatigue

· changes in emotional status or behavior

· changes in sensory, motor, or nervous system functioning

· insomnia or sleep problems

· a parent's feeling that his or her child "just isn't right"

longer than fifteen minutes, and may include amnesia. In this archaic form of grading, only athletes who blacked out, whether for mere seconds or a more prolonged period of time, were worthy of a grade 3 "severe" classification.

It's not really hard to understand why for so long, loss of consciousness was considered an appropriate indicator of the severity of a concussion. After all, when an athlete has actually been knocked out, even if only for a few seconds, it just *seems* like a more serious injury than one that leaves the athlete feeling only a little dazed. Yet that's just not the case—loss of consciousness alone is not a reliable predictor of the severity of concussion or the projected length of time needed to recover.[4] And in fact, loss of consciousness occurs in only about one of every ten concussions.[5] Though all symptoms are important and noteworthy, more recent research has suggested that amnesia may actually be the better predictor of the road ahead; athletes who experience amnesia after a head injury tend to have longer and more problematic recovery periods.[6] (Amnesia, by the way, can be described as *retrograde* or *anterograde*. Retrograde amnesia means the athlete can't recall events that occurred before the injury, and anterograde means the athlete can't recall events immediately following the injury.)

Another problem with relying on these kinds of arbitrary grading systems is that proper classification is contingent on an athlete's willingness and ability to properly and accurately self-report symptoms. For example, a loss of consciousness or extreme trouble maintaining one's balance may be obvious to observant bystanders; the athlete herself doesn't have to confirm the presence of these symptoms. But only the concussed athlete can identify and describe symptoms such as headache, blurred vision, nausea, dizziness, and numbness or tingling in the extremities. If the athlete doesn't think an injury is serious enough to warrant attention or doesn't want to ride the bench for the remainder of the game, she may be inclined to underplay the existence of any symptoms, or not report them at all. (So much for using a measure of reported symptoms to determine the severity of the injury!) There is widespread belief among medical professionals that athletes should not be returned to play after a suspected concussion, based solely on the likelihood that self-reporting is unreliable.[7]

But perhaps the biggest problem with these kinds of grading systems is that for so long they were used to determine how long an athlete should be removed from play, and when it was "safe" to return to the sport. For example, the 1997 American Academy of Neurology classification system I mentioned earlier proposed the following return-to-play guidelines, which are now outdated: same-day return to play for a grade 1 (mild) concussion; one week without sports for multiple grade 1 concussions, a grade 2 (moderate), or a grade 3 concussion where the athlete blacked out only briefly; two weeks without sports for multiple grade

The King-Devick Test: Accurate Post-Concussion Sideline Screening?

New research published in the medical journal *Neurology* has suggested that the King-Devick test, a 1980s-era reading and vision test developed by optometrists Al King and Steve Devick, may have some use as a rapid, accurate sideline screening for athletes with a suspected concussion.[9] The test, which requires athletes to read a series of single-digit numbers on a timed basis, takes only two minutes to complete and does not require a medical professional to administer. It has been suggested that athletes who read the numbers at a slower pace than their baseline reading test should be removed from play and referred for medical evaluation by a doctor. Early advocates have surmised that the King-Devick may become *the* standard sideline test for sports-related concussions.

Though the King-Devick may prove to be a great addition to the sideline tool set, it's important to remember that the best way to measure and diagnose a concussion is by testing a *variety* of skills. For example, I might see a concussed athlete demonstrate strong reaction time on post-concussion testing but show weak verbal or design memory. It's also possible for symptoms of concussion to appear days after impact. So no matter how "well" your child performs on a sideline assessment test—no matter what type of test is being used—he or she should not be returned to play until examined by a licensed health care professional.[10]

2 concussions or a grade 3 with a more prolonged loss of consciousness (minutes rather than seconds); and one month or longer without sports for multiple grade 3 concussions.

Arbitrary guidelines such as these may be misinterpreted to mean that the day-counting begins with the date of injury rather than the day when concussion symptoms subside. For example, if a grade 2 injury occurred during a Friday night game, and the athlete didn't begin to experience full symptoms until Monday morning, you can see how a one-week period of rest may not be enough time for the athlete's brain to completely heal. (In fact, studies show that high school athletes in particular often exhibit significant memory deficits—meaning they are still technically exhibiting symptoms—on day eight following an injury. Prescribing seven days of rest after the injury date, then, would be insufficient.)[8] Any type of symptom may be a sign that the brain is still in a state of metabolic slowdown or "depression," making it that much more vulnerable to sustaining a second, far more severe injury, such as second impact syndrome. You can see, then, why arbitrary guidelines like "one week without sports" can be so potentially dangerous.

As of this writing, there are no research- or evidence-based guidelines or formulae for determining how long an athlete should stay off the playing field, especially in the case of child athletes. These days, we judge the severity of a concussion after the athlete feels asymptomatic (is no longer experiencing symptoms), has been examined by a medical professional, has been given time to rest, and has demonstrated improvement on post-concussion cognitive and physical exertional testing (see Chapters 4 and 5 for more on physical exertional testing). In other words, you can't determine how serious a concussion is until after the athlete has recovered. This is why no athlete with symptoms should ever be allowed to return to play. When in doubt, sit them out! (Brain injury expert Robert Cantu, MD, is generally credited with introducing this now-popular concussion education phrase.)

THE LINGERING EFFECTS OF POST-CONCUSSION SYNDROME

For some athletes, kicking the symptoms of concussion may not be easy, especially if the athlete did not seek immediate mental and physical rest following injury, did not take time off from the sport, or has a history of multiple concussions. When symptoms linger for weeks (or even months) on end, post-concussion syndrome (PCS) is to blame. The symptoms of PCS can be grouped into four general categories: (1) physical; (2) emotional/behavioral (for example, depression or anxiety); (3) cognitive (difficulty concentrating or increased forgetfulness); and (4) sleep related.

Post-concussion syndrome is more or less what it sounds like: it's the prolonged presence of concussion-related symptoms, usually lasting from one to three months after the injury, or even longer. (Some physicians will diagnose PCS if symptoms have lasted for at least three months with no full recovery; more recently, concussion experts have begun diagnosing PCS if the athlete still has symptoms one month after the injury was sustained.) There's plenty we still don't know about PCS, but we do know that children who are not given adequate time to rest, sleep, and heal after an injury are much more likely to develop PCS, and to suffer from it for longer periods of time. In fact, studies of high school students have shown that athletes who were allowed to rest after injury recovered twice as quickly as those who were not.[11]

Unfortunately, many symptoms of PCS are "unseen" and cognitive in nature, so they routinely go unnoticed. Ongoing cognitive symptoms, including problems with multitasking; an increase in errors on tests and homework; distractibility and problems with attention and focus; forgetfulness; problems following busy conversations; and confusion in noisy, high-stimulus environments, are all symptoms of PCS. However, they are also symptoms that are difficult to diagnose or pinpoint outright. It's hard to tell, for example, if your child has simply flubbed a test or two, or if he's actually suffering from the residual effects of brain injury, *especially* if you didn't even know he sustained a concussion in the first place.

In Chapter 1, I explained that the brain requires an immense amount of energy to function, but that concussions trigger an energy *depletion*—this is why people with concussions tend to feel sluggish or fuzzy; essentially, their brains are just really, really tired. Therefore, if you send a child back to school with a case of undiagnosed PCS, you're inadvertently putting a lot of stress on an already overtaxed brain. Engaging in even the most basic cognitive functions, the kinds of tasks that children and adolescents perform every single day—from paying attention in class, to doing math homework, to text messaging friends, to playing elaborate video games—may actually prolong the recovery process or cause a gradual worsening of symptoms. This is why children suffering from PCS may experience an unexpected and unexplained decline in grades, increasing episodes of incomplete homework assignments, or an increase in behavioral problems.

If those symptoms seem to have appeared out of the blue, yet persist long enough, concerned and confused parents typically start looking for some kind of explanation. Children with undiagnosed concussions can sometimes be misdiagnosed with attention deficit hyperactivity disorder (ADHD) or with a learning disorder; I've seen this more than once in my own office. A child with no history of academic or behavioral difficulties might come in for testing to diagnose a learning disorder, but I'll be able to trace the symptoms back to an overlooked brain injury. These kinds of misdiagnoses can wound a child's sense of self, alter his or her academic career, and cut short athletic endeavors. In short, misdiagnosis can be devastating. To prevent these kinds of misdiagnoses, any out-of-character changes in your child athlete's cognitive abilities, emotional behaviors, physical symptoms, or sleep patterns should prompt a thorough examination for the possibility of PCS.

COULD A SIMPLE BLOOD TEST ACCURATELY DIAGNOSE A CONCUSSION?

You may remember hearing about the untimely death of Tony Award–winning actress Natasha Richardson in March 2009. After falling and hitting her head during a beginners' skiing lesson at a resort in Quebec, Canada, the actress twice refused medical attention—after all, she'd only slipped, she was talking and acting normally, and she claimed that she felt fine—only to develop an undiagnosed epidural hematoma (brain bleed) and die two days later. The tragedy left people everywhere wondering: how could a simple fall turn into such a devastating injury? Could her life have been saved if we'd known what to look for? She was only forty-five years old.

We've learned that concussions and other brain injuries are often difficult to detect, and that undiagnosed and untreated brain injuries can lead to serious and long-term consequences—from PCS, to a greater like-

> ## The Four Categories of Post-Concussion Syndrome Symptoms
>
> *Cognitive:* the athlete exhibits problems with attention, concentration, memory and learning, mental processing and speed, reaction time
>
> *Emotional/Behavioral:* irritability, sadness, depression, anxiety, nervousness, anger, emotional instability
>
> *Physical:* headache, sensitivity to light and sound, balance problems, numbness, fatigue, nausea, changes in appetite
>
> *Sleep:* insomnia, sleepiness, drowsiness, sleeping more or less than usual

lihood of suffering sis, to brain damage or dementia, to CTE and even death. Because of this, medical researchers have been attempting to develop some sort of simple blood test to accurately and definitively diagnose concussions and other forms of traumatic brain injury. This kind of testing is already utilized in the treatment of cardiac patients: if you are sent to the hospital with chest pains, for example, your doctor may order a *troponin test.* Troponin is a kind of protein that the heart muscle releases into the bloodstream when it's injured. Because healthy people do not have troponin floating around in their blood, the presence of troponin is a good indication that the patient is, indeed, suffering from a heart attack. At present, the troponin test is just one tool that doctors use to help make their diagnoses. Cardiologists may also order an electrocardiogram (EKG) to monitor the beating of the heart, or an angiogram, to monitor blockages and plaque buildup in the arteries.

Troponin is an example of a *biomarker,* a chemical or protein that marks, or indicates, a particular biological state. It's also not the only biomarker that may be associated with heart attacks. Troponin indicates damage to the heart muscle itself, but researchers are currently attempting to discover other biomarkers that might be present when, say, blood flow to the heart muscle is reduced; this would enable doctors to detect a heart condition long before the muscle itself is damaged or dying. The hope for the treatment of concussions is that researchers will be able to isolate one or several biomarkers that appear in the bloodstream when a person has sustained a brain injury. If the research proves successful, a simple blood test would take all the guesswork out of diagnosing concussions. And that kind of medical breakthrough would have amazing implications, from less money spent on expensive (but less accurate) tests such as CT scans, to a lesser chance that brain injuries will go undiagnosed and untreated.

The American military, in particular, is quite interested in this kind of diagnostic development. Brain injuries have become one of the most common wounds among soldiers fighting in Iraq and Afghanistan, due mainly to blasts and explosions from roadside bombs or improvised explosive devices (IEDs)—it's estimated that more than 350,000 American soldiers, roughly 20 percent of those deployed, have sustained a serious brain injury while in combat.[12] However, it's incredibly difficult to diagnose a concussion in the field. That's largely why the military has already funneled about $1.7 billion into brain injury research since 2007.[13, 14] And in October 2010, the US Department of Defense (DOD) awarded a $26.3 million contract to Banyan Biomarkers, Inc., a privately held medical research company, to develop a diagnostic blood test as well as prototypes of portable testing devices that could be used in combat.[15] "You can't bring a CAT scan machine up a mountain in Afghanistan," Jackson Streeter, MD, chief medical officer for Banyan Biomarkers, told *ESPN The Magazine*. "That's why the Army is interested."[16]

Although the Banyan Biomarkers research is some of the most promising, most of the focus has been on hospitalized patients with more severe brain injuries, a population that differs from athletes with concussions; it's still not clear whether these types of tests will be capable of detecting more "mild" brain injuries. (The contract with DOD will fund a clinical trial of 1,200 patients to determine if the blood test is reliable and accurate; that trial is scheduled to conclude sometime in 2013. The test would then have to be submitted for FDA approval.) It's perhaps not surprising that some scientists and other experts are still quite skeptical. Yet traumatic brain injury research is such a rapidly evolving field of medicine, it's possible that such a test could be available within the next few years. This kind of "point-of-care" blood test could become the first step in determining safe and universal guidelines for making return-to-play decisions, something doctors have been attempting to do for decades. Though it's most likely that no single stand-alone test will be able to determine when recovery from concussion has occurred, for now all we can do is wait.

EARLY IDENTIFICATION OF CONCUSSION SPEEDS RECOVERY

Brain injury specialists now know that identifying a concussion early and managing it properly—by prescribing an adequate period of rest—can decrease the recovery period, reduce lasting effects, lessen the probability of developing PCS, and help athletes and their parents make safe return-to-play decisions. In short, concussions need to be taken seriously. And because even basic, everyday academic endeavors like homework assignments and tests require lots of energy from the brain, "adequate rest" may even include missing a few days of school and receiving special academic accommodations, such as no homework for a short time and the rescheduling or postponement of tests and quizzes. Unfortunately, many students—particularly high achievers—as well as parents and school officials balk at these types of recommendations for rest and medical leave, especially those who are not up to date on the most recent concussion research and guidelines. Yet we see that athletes who are given the chance to rest will recover much more quickly than those who immediately return to their normal daily routines. If your child sustains a concussion, you may need to ask yourself this simple question: is it better for her to miss a few days of school now, or to potentially struggle with concentration, focus, memory, and behavioral problems for months on end? Sometimes kids, and their parents, need a bit of a reality check.

Speaking of reality checks, it's extremely important to educate your children on the signs and symptoms of brain injury. It is never safe to

Case Study No. 1

PATIENT: Jason, twelve-year-old male

PREFERRED SPORT(S): Basketball (elite private travel league); soccer

FIRST APPOINTMENT WITH DR. MOSER: February 2011

TYPE OF AND DATE(S) OF INJURY: Age eleven. During a recreation league basketball game, Jason was closely guarding another player when their heads collided; Jason was hit square in the nose. *Immediate symptoms*: Lethargy, confusion, teary eyes, seemed "out of sorts." Jason's father encouraged the coach to remove Jason from the game.

The following morning, Tuesday, Jason woke up with a headache, so his mother kept him home from school. On Wednesday and Thursday Jason seemed fine. But by Thursday night, after playing in another basketball game, his headache had returned. He was taken to his pediatrician on Friday morning. Despite the lingering headache, Jason's doctor didn't seem overly concerned about the situation. He did not order any tests, and there was no discussion about the need for mental and physical rest, or about the danger of returning a concussed child back to sports too soon. The doctor sent Jason home, telling his parents he'd be "fine." Jason's parents were skeptical, and when their son's headache persisted, they brought him to my concussion center.

INITIAL EXAM: Though his pediatrician hadn't seemed too concerned, Jason's lingering headache was a sign that he *had* sustained a concussion, and that his brain had not yet healed. I had him sit for post-concussion neurocognitive testing (specifically, ImPACT testing; read more about this in the next chapter). Because he had never had a preseason baseline established, I had Jason repeat the testing process during several follow-up appointments, to help determine when he had recovered and when it would be safe for him to return to play.

RECOVERY PLAN: Complete mental and physical rest: no computer, no reading, no chores, no exercise, no video games, no birthday parties, no socializing. Mild television; lots of extra sleep. Jason stayed home from school for one week, until his headaches were gone and his post-concussion neurocognitive test scores had improved. And to be on the safe side, Jason sat out from sports for three weeks after his symptoms had subsided.

NOTES: Jason's case shows us that even though your child may *seem* fine a few days after a concussion, symptoms can reappear (and often do!) especially if the child returns to school and sports without having completed an appropriate course of rest. Remember, recurring or lingering symptoms are signs that the brain has not yet fully healed, and is therefore vulnerable to a second, potentially much more serious injury. Luckily, Jason's parents knew enough to seek out a second opinion. Once Jason was allowed to rest and recover, his injury healed and his symptoms went away. Today, he's a healthy, happy seventh grader.

NOTES FROM JASON'S DAD: "Even though my wife and I were both in the stands when Jason got his concussion, my wife didn't even see the impact—it happened in the blink of an eye. Which just goes to show you, you can't always rely on someone else to notice when your child gets hurt. Coaches usually have a lot on their mind, between running a game and making player substitutions; it's not possible for them to watch every player every second of the game. And though I know lots of parents who drop their children off at practices and games, and pick them up when the workout is over, I think it's imperative to be there for your child, looking out for his or her safety. I knew immediately that something wasn't right with Jason after he got hit in the nose. A more subtle collision, however, would be much easier to miss.

"For the first few weeks after his return to play, I could tell that Jason had lost some of his confidence on the court, he was much more cautious, and much more concerned about getting injured again. But the good thing that's come out of our experience is that I know, without a doubt, that Jason will be honest with me if he were to sustain another concussion. He understands now that concussions have to be taken seriously, and that you have to protect your brain."

assume that children know what to look for, or that they understand the long-term consequences of concussions. And in fact, research indicates that the majority of children do not. In a study of more than 1,500 high school students, for example, 66.4 percent of those who had sustained a concussion did not think their symptoms were "serious enough" to report. And 41 percent did not report their symptoms because they "did not want to leave the game." Just over 36 percent did not even realize that they had sustained a probable concussion, based on their symptoms at the time of injury.[17]

Sit down with your child and talk about the symptoms of concussion (use the chart on page 37 if you need a refresher). Make sure he understands that if he has a headache, or feels fuzzy, or just doesn't feel *right*, he needs to take a break and tell an adult. Explain that, yes, if he gets a concussion, he may have to sit out for a while. But if he *ignores* a concussion, because he doesn't think it's serious or because he doesn't want to ride the bench, he might have trouble in school, or lasting symptoms, or—worst-case scenario—have to stop playing the sport he loves altogether. The earlier you identify the signs of a concussion, the faster you can get your child back out on the field. And it's always better to be safe than sorry.

Chapter 2 Review

- The presence of *any* single sign or symptom is enough to suspect a concussion. When in doubt, sit them out!

- Post-concussion syndrome, or PCS, occurs when symptoms linger for weeks. If your child athlete exhibits changes in behavior or sleep patterns, or complains of physical or emotional symptoms, seek an immediate medical evaluation to rule out a brain injury.

- Teach your children how to identify the signs and symptoms of concussion. Don't assume that they already know what to watch for, or that they understand the severity and long-term consequences of brain injuries.

· Early identification of concussion speeds recovery. If you suspect a brain injury, don't wait to seek medical treatment. Start your child on an immediate course of mental and physical rest.

THE BEST OFFENSE IS A GOOD DEFENSE
Preseason Baseline Testing

Despite all the dangers associated with mild traumatic brain injury (mTBI), concussions are not something we can fully prevent. Even if you were to forbid your child to play sports, kids are not immune to slips and trips, falling off a bike, tumbling from a skateboard, or the risk of injury in more serious, spontaneous events, such as a sudden car crash or freak accident. (As I mentioned in Chapter 1, very young children are actually more likely to sustain a head injury during recess or free play than while participating in organized athletics.) We just can't protect our children from every possible circumstance; we can't protect them from every possible injury—even though, as parents, we often try. Still, you may be wondering if there's anything you can do to protect your child *before* a concussion occurs. Is there any way to be proactive? The answer is yes.

In the 1980s, a neuropsychologist at the University of Virginia, Dr. Jeffrey Barth, had the brilliant notion that it might be possible to track recovery from sports-related concussion by measuring brain performance both *before* and *after* an athlete sustained a brain injury. Neurocognitive preseason (or baseline) testing was born. How it works is simple: first, a healthy athlete is tested to measure basic brain-based cognitive skills. Later, if he or she sustains a concussion, the athlete is retested and the scores are compared. Once healed, athletes are expected to perform at least as well as—or preferably better than—their baseline test scores before being allowed to return to play.[1]

This kind of neurocognitive testing (interchangeably referred to as neuro*psychological* testing) is particularly useful because it can identify lingering cognitive symptoms, such as slower reaction time or problems with memory, that are often difficult to detect. For example, your child may feel fine a few days after a rough tackle—his headaches might have subsided, or his vision may no longer be blurred—but testing may reveal that his brain is still functioning a little slower than usual, that his injury has not yet fully healed. Because we know that allowing a young athlete to return to sports too soon puts him or her at risk of developing post-concussion syndrome or second impact syndrome (a potentially fatal condition), baseline testing can offer a certain added measure of safety. Neurocognitive testing is also effective because it can identify symptoms that an athlete may be unwilling or unable to admit. (We already know that children—and adults—might be tempted to downplay the severity of their symptoms, just so they can get back to practice.)

In the next chapter I'll provide you with a detailed, step-by-step plan to follow if you suspect your child has sustained a concussion. But in this chapter, I'll focus more specifically on the pre-concussion testing procedure itself. (Post-concussion testing requires greater clinical expertise and should ideally be performed by a neuropsychologist. We'll talk more about that later, too.) What's important to understand at the outset is that neurocognitive testing is not *diagnostic*, meaning that it cannot be used to definitively determine if a concussion has occurred, and it shouldn't be the *only* tool that doctors use to determine when an athlete may return to play. Also, neurocognitive testing should not be confused with sideline testing, which is performed immediately after an injury is sustained, in order to determine how oriented the athlete is and to document his or her *immediate* symptoms. Nor should neurocognitive testing be confused with or used in place of a medical assessment. If you think your child has sustained a concussion, he or she should be evaluated by a physician to rule out a more serious (or potentially life-threatening) injury, such as a skull fracture or brain hemorrhage.

BASELINE TESTING, PAST AND PRESENT

The concept of preseason baseline concussion testing was born out of traditional neuropsychological testing. Neuropsychologists—doctors who are brain behavior specialists—are trained to identify and diagnose brain disorders, brain diseases, and brain injury. To do so, they typically measure the patient's cognitive abilities using a long series of paper-pencil tests, which are comprehensive but time-consuming. At the time of Dr. Barth's 1980s-era study of college football players, such tests weren't practical for the diagnosis and treatment of concussion: it might take hours to complete a single battery of tests, and the results might not be available for up to a week or even longer—not exactly helpful when, in many cases, the symptoms of concussion may have subsided by then. So Barth worked to develop a short series of tests that targeted the specific types of cognitive functions that are most often affected by a sports-related concussion, and that could be administered easily, efficiently, and repeatedly. (In a post-concussion follow-up, the athlete is tested serially —or repeatedly—until reaching his or her own baseline. So that possible "practice effects," or improvement in scores from having taken the same test over and over, are not confused with a real healing of the brain injury, most post-concussion exams are available in several, slightly different versions. That way, the athlete doesn't take the same test again in sequence.)

A decade or so after Barth's research, neuropsychologists working with the National Hockey League developed another short battery of tests that looked at a wide variety of brain functions, such as attention, concentration, memory, and reaction time. But back then, it still took at least forty-five minutes to test each individual athlete on a team, and a neuropsychologist had to be available to administer the test. The obvious need for even greater efficiency eventually led to the creation of computerized pre- and post-concussion baseline testing. Computerized tests could be completed in just twenty or thirty minutes, making it possible to baseline many athletes, including entire sports teams, simultaneously in a computer lab, and to do so without the actual presence of a neuropsychologist. Instead, a trained technician or athletic trainer could administer baselines, with training and oversight from a neuropsychologist. "I used to sit across from athletes doing paper-and-pencil memory tests," Dr. Mark Lovell, former director of neuropsychological testing for the NFL, told *Time* magazine in 2011. "That would never [have worked] with large groups of kids. There aren't that many neuropsychologists alive."[2] Once the tests were computerized, doctors could easily baseline large numbers of athletes (and eventually student or youth athletes) with just a few laptops.

These days, most professional sports leagues, including the NHL, NFL, MLB (Major League Baseball), and NASCAR, have an official league-wide baseline testing program in place. Because this type of neuropsychological testing was designed specifically to identify changes in cognitive ability, the kinds of brain function most affected by concussion, we know that it is more sensitive to—and therefore more effective at—monitoring concussions than are neurological or radiological testing (such as CT scans or MRIs). It makes sense, then, that concussion-testing programs, similar to those employed at the professional level, are springing up in colleges and high schools across the country.[3]

NEUROCOGNITIVE TESTING TODAY

Currently, there are four major computerized neurocognitive concussion tests on the market:

- Automated Neuropsychological Assessment Metrics (ANAM)
- Axon Sports Computerized Cognitive Assessment Tool (formerly known as CogSport)
- HeadMinder Concussion Resolution Index
- Immediate Post-Concussion Assessment and Cognitive Test (ImPACT)

Each of these tests has its own advantages and disadvantages, but in the interest of full disclosure, I am a credentialed IMPACT provider, I have conducted and published research on IMPACT testing, and I use IMPACT testing in my clinical practice. Though some other tests are growing in popularity, IMPACT is still the most widely used among both professional and amateur sports teams, and is likely the most researched and critiqued of all the neurocognitive tests available. For all of these reasons, I will focus specifically on IMPACT testing in the remainder of this chapter.

IMPACT consists of six short neuropsychological tests, designed to target different aspects of cognitive function, including attention, visual memory, visual-motor (or processing) speed, and reaction time. Just to give you an idea of the types of questions and tasks that make up IMPACT, here's a brief explanation of the first test, which measures attention by way of verbal recognition:

A series of twelve "target words" flash briefly on the computer screen. Then, the athlete is shown a list of twenty-four words, twelve of which are target words and twelve of which are not. The athlete is asked to remember and identify which are the target words from the original list of twelve. Just to make things a little more complicated, the non-target words are quite similar to the target words—so if the target word is *hill*, for instance, the non-target word might be *mountain*. Obviously, the athlete has to be paying pretty close attention to get the answers right.[4]

From these six short neuropsychological tests, five separate composite scores are generated: (1) verbal memory, (2) visual memory, (3) visual motor speed, (4) reaction time, and (5) impulse control. IMPACT also includes a symptom checklist, which allows the individual to rate each of his or her symptoms on a 0-to-6 scale. Once the athlete has completed the test, the IMPACT company provides an immediate, detailed report of the scores, including the percentage of answers the athlete got correct, as well as scores in the form of percentiles. So, not unlike SAT or statewide achievement testing, you can see where your athlete ranks among other children in his or her age group. (A 50th percentile score would be considered average and normal; it means that of 100 people of the same age and gender, the student is approximately stronger in test performance than 50 of them.) The IMPACT program also stores all of the athlete's previous test scores in a database, so pre- and post-concussion results can be easily compared.

I have often heard parents of a concussed athlete tell me that their child "failed the test." But baseline testing is not a pass/fail scenario. It is not intelligence or achievement testing, nor can it be used to diagnose learning, attention, or other brain disorders. Rather, baseline testing is simply a screening tool; it provides a snapshot of how a particular individual functions at a specific time (like before an injury occurs). Later, serial or repeated testing is performed to help determine when the athlete has fully recovered. There are cases in which a student may recover, but may never return to her baseline. There are also cases in which a student's post-concussion test looks fine, but he still has physical symptoms, such as a persistent headache (the presence of any unresolved symptom indicates that he has not yet fully healed, or that there may be something else going on medically).

All of these variations mean that each concussion is unique, and each must be treated individually. You can't compare one person's concussion to another's. The reason that IMPACT provides *percentile* reporting (allowing you to see where your child ranks among others of a similar age) is that percentile reporting is helpful if your child never had a baseline established in the first place. So, even if your child never underwent baseline testing, you can still take her in for post-concussion testing. The neuropsychologist or other neurocognitive concussion specialist will then use percentile scores to gauge if she is performing within the range that is estimated to be normal for her, and will have her take the post-concussion test several times during the course of recovery to check for improvement. (Of course, without a baseline on file, it's impossible to know if, prior to the injury, your child would typically have scored in the 50th percentile [average range] or the 90th percentile [well above average]).

Computerized IMPACT testing may be found in two different versions: the older, desktop computer version (which some schools and organizations still use), and the newer test, which is available online. Though the tests are nearly identical, there are some important distinctions:

1. The online version has updated "norms" based on a larger pool of people, spanning a larger age range.

2. The online test can be accessed from any computer with an Internet connection (as opposed to the desktop version, which requires a specific software package).

3. The desktop version requires the athlete to use both left and right mouse clicks (using either the index or middle finger) to indicate answers to certain questions, including timed-reaction questions. Research shows us, however, that individuals tend to favor their index finger over the middle finger, and this left-right confusion can lead to incorrect, if unintended, responses. In order to lessen this chance of error, the online version of the test uses the keyboard instead of a mouse for certain parts of the test.[5]

4. The online version offers a better-quality printed score report (with helpful visual graphics).

5. The online version computes the Cognitive Efficiency Index, which measures the relationship between the athlete's accuracy in answering the questions and the speed at which he or she responds. The desktop version has no Cognitive Efficiency Index.

6. The online version automatically flags "suspicious" scores (for example, when a child does not put forth his or her best effort), whereas the desktop version does not.

7. Tests taken online are stored by the IMPACT company. The desktop version, on the other hand, does not require an Internet connection, so the data is stored by the owner of the software (typically the school or concussion center).

I've used both versions of IMPACT in my clinical practice, but these days, most schools and sports concussion treatment centers employ the up-

> ## Did You Know . . . ?
>
> Baseline test scores should be reviewed by a trained specialist to ensure that they are accurate and true. Several factors, such as distraction in the testing room, confusion about the test instructions, or faulty computer equipment, could trigger an invalid baseline score. Post-concussion tests require even more clinical expertise for interpretation. Neuropsychologists, in particular, understand the various factors that may affect test performance and are best trained to interpret post-concussion testing.

dated online version. It's important to point out that there can be a mild difference in scores between the desktop and online versions. If your child took a baseline test on the desktop version, for example, and the school then updated its concussion-testing software, and your child later took a post-concussion test using the newer, online version, there could be some discrepancy in percentile scoring—it's sort of like trying to compare Red Delicious and McIntosh apples. So, in the best-case scenario, pre- and post-concussion testing should be performed using the same version of the test. (If the school or concussion treatment center upgrades its software, it might be helpful to have your child take the test again and have a new baseline established. In my own clinical research, I've discovered that the online test tends to produce slightly more valid scores than does the older, desktop version.) Likewise, pre- and post-concussion testing should be performed using the same test *brand*. A baseline test using Im-PACT, for example, and a post-concussion test performed with Axon or HeadMinder can't easily be compared; they're different tests.

ENSURING THE VALIDITY OF COMPUTERIZED BASELINE SCORES: WHAT TEST ADMINISTRATORS AND PARENTS NEED TO KNOW

If the entire point of baseline testing is to help make a more informed decision about when an athlete should be allowed to return to play—if the entire point is to ensure an athlete's health and safety—then it makes sense to take all the necessary steps to ensure that the baseline test is an accurate depiction of the athlete's true cognitive ability. In short, you want to make sure your child's baseline test is *valid*. But baseline testing isn't a perfect science, and there are things that both parents and test interpreters alike should understand about the way baseline testing is often performed.

Most middle schools, high schools, and even most universities do not have a trained neuropsychologist or other neurocognitive specialist on staff. So baseline testing programs like IMPACT are typically purchased by the school and administered to large groups of students—for example, an entire football team—by a nurse or certified athletic trainer. On some level, that makes perfect sense. After all, testing large groups of students at one time requires less staffing, and is therefore both cost- and time-efficient. However, many school administrators and athletic personnel don't realize that baseline tests need to be administered under the supervision and guidance of a neurocognitive specialist. They assume that students can be corralled to take the baseline test, and that the scores can be stored in the computer and not looked at until a concussion occurs. Unfortunately, that's just not the case. Several extraneous factors can trigger an invalid or inaccurate baseline test:

> · *Lack of motivation.* In some cases, the athlete may just not "feel like" taking the test, or may not be "in the mood." This can often be attributed to a lack of education about the importance of the test. If the athlete doesn't understand why the testing is being performed, or how the testing works, or why she needs to try her best (in order to ensure an accurate, valid score), she may be inclined to answer haphazardly or randomly, just to get the thing over with. This is why I recommend explaining the procedure and the importance of baseline testing to children before they even reach the testing site. The more they understand, the more likely they'll be to stay focused.

> **Did You Know . . . ?**
>
> Athletes may try to perform poorly on baseline testing on purpose, so that after sustaining an injury, their post-concussion scores won't look so bad by comparison. Unfortunately, this kind of behavior can only hurt an athlete's chance for a speedy return to play. Very low baseline scores are a red flag to the concussion doctor that the test may have been invalid or inaccurate; in such a case, after a concussion, the doctor will be forced to order repeated testing, keeping the athlete off the field for even longer than may be necessary.

· *"Sandbagging."* There is widespread speculation among concussion specialists that some athletes might be inclined to underperform on a baseline test—on *purpose*—so that if they were made to take a *post*-concussion test, they would perform comparatively better and therefore be allowed to return to play sooner. It's also thought that some students might purposely perform poorly on a post-concussion test in order to reap some kind of benefit—for example, ensuring a longer medical leave or enjoying a longer period of academic accommodation (less homework and no tests). In other words, some kids could choose to "fake it."[6–13]

Trying to prevent intentional sandbagging is incredibly difficult for test administrators (not to mention parents). After all, how do you force a kid to take a test he doesn't want to take, and how would you even know if he had tanked the test on purpose? This is one reason that the online version of IMPACT is programmed to automatically flag test protocols that seem suspicious. One of those flags is an elevated Impulse Control Composite score. For example, IMPACT features a number of timed response questions, meaning the athlete is asked to answer as quickly as he can. But if he answers too quickly—or faster than would be considered possible or feasible—the test will be flagged as suspicious, and his Impulse Control score will go up. An Impulse Control score higher than 30 would indicate that an athlete may be answering randomly, rather than taking his time and answering to the best of his ability. In instances where the Impulse Control score is high, the test should be discarded and readministered. Studies indicate that somewhere between 2 percent and 9 percent of high school athletes, and about 5 percent of college athletes, may return an invalid test based on an elevated Impulse Control score.[14, 15] There are other types of red flags or "invalidity factors" besides the Impulse Control score, but they all are meant to alert the test interpreter to check for validity. If the baseline scores are never reviewed, though, then the flags become useless.

· *Environmental factors.* Imagine that your child is one of thirty or forty players on a high school football team. Now imagine that roughly half of that entire, rowdy team of adolescent boys is crowded into a quiet computer lab, seated side by side, and made to take a test that measures focus, attention, memory, and reaction time. What's the likelihood that your child will *not* be distracted by squeaking chairs, random coughs, muffled laughter, or back-of-the-room whispering? What's the likelihood that his baseline test will be a true and accurate reflection of his abilities?

Unfortunately, baseline testing is often performed this way, in a group setting in a computer lab where the chance of distraction is quite high. (As I mentioned earlier, it's typically cheaper and easier for the school to churn through testing in this manner.) Further complicating matters is the fact that *post*-concussion testing is not generally performed in a group setting—it's not as if an entire football team will have suffered a collective concussion and need to be evaluated all together. Post-concussion testing, therefore, is usually performed in a quiet, distraction-free room, and the athlete is alone. Because the whole point is to compare post-concussion test results with baseline results, it's important to try to limit the chance of distraction or interruption as much as possible during baseline testing. Think about it: your child's post-concussion test might compare favorably with her baseline test, simply because she was better able to concentrate. It might appear that her testing has improved, when really she just wasn't as distracted the second time around. This discrepancy could contribute to an earlier—but riskier—return to play, defeating the entire purpose of the testing.

There are several ways for schools and testing centers to control the testing environment and experience, including providing seating that is comfortably spaced (athletes should not be seated too close to each other or across from one another); using soundproofing or white-noise machines to drown out extraneous sounds or interruptions; providing clear group instructions regarding communication during testing (instructing students to raise their hands with questions or problems); having one or two trained test administrators present *at all times*; identifying and removing an athlete who is overly talkative or disruptive, and testing him or her later individually; and testing when fatigue is not an issue (ideally, testing should not be performed at the end of a long day or immediately following exercise, practice, or a game).

Research that my colleagues and I conducted shows us that somewhere between 6 percent and 11 percent of high school athletes may wind up with an invalid baseline test for one reason or another.[16] Although that's not an incredibly high percentage (especially when compared with other kinds of neurocognitive data), you can see now why it's so important for baseline test scores to be reviewed for accuracy. Unfortunately, this aspect of quality assurance is often overlooked in large schools that test athletes en masse. In fact, in a recent survey of 399 athletic trainers at various high schools, colleges, and universities, 95 percent of respondents reported using IMPACT for baseline testing, but only 54.8% actually examined the validity of those results.[17] Even though a suspicious IMPACT test may be automatically flagged, without a review of the scores, it's unlikely that the test will be identified as invalid, or that the athlete in question will be asked to retake the test.

Aside from the need to review baseline tests for validity in general, it's important to note that baseline and post-concussion tests should be reviewed by a trained neurocognitive specialist, specifically. Neuropsychologists are the best qualified to interpret testing, especially when evaluating an athlete with a history of ADHD, a learning or mental disorder, or a history of multiple concussions. Neuropsychologists have been trained to recognize and understand additional factors that might affect performance, including test anxiety, sleep difficulties, medications, or drug and alcohol use. When there is no baseline available for comparison, a neuropsychologist can interpret serial (or repeated) post-concussion tests to help determine when the athlete has likely recovered and is ready to return to play. If we're going to provide computerized testing programs in our schools, then it's imperative that those programs be administered in the most effective manner possible. The value of baseline and post-concussion testing really depends on the knowledge and diligence of the test administrator and the interpreter.

WHY ALL PARENTS SHOULD PERIODICALLY UPDATE THEIR CHILD'S CONCUSSION BASELINE

Even though baseline testing is meant to be performed before an injury occurs, it shouldn't be thought of as a one-time thing. For example, if your child sustained a concussion at age eighteen, but hadn't been baseline tested since age twelve, you'd be attempting to compare the cognitive abilities of a high school senior to a seventh grader, an inaccurate comparison to be sure. As parents well know, children can have considerable growth spurts in a single year. And just as they grow bigger and taller, their cognitive brain structures grow and mature as well.

Although some experts advocate testing as often as every six months, many concussion experts—myself included—recommend updating baseline test results on a yearly basis. This kind of repetitive baseline testing can not only anticipate maturational growth spurts, but it can also take into account mild concussions that might have gone unnoticed or undiagnosed, as well as cumulative deficits from a series of unreported subconcussive blows (blows that aren't strong enough to trigger immediate symptoms, but that may cause problems over time). Unfortunately, yearly testing can be expensive and time-consuming, and many schools may not consider it practical. We'll talk more about how to secure private baseline testing in the next chapter.

When and if a child sustains a concussion, she will be retested, typically a few times during the recovery period, to determine when her cognitive functioning has returned to normal, when she's fully healed, and when she can safely return to playing sports. As with baseline testing, experts vary in their recommendations for when, following an injury, to begin post-concussion testing and how often to repeat it. Some experts believe that as long as the athlete has a baseline score on file, she shouldn't be tested at all following a concussion until all of her symptoms have subsided. Others believe that getting a cognitive snapshot of the athlete within a twenty-four- to forty-eight-hour window following an injury can help determine the severity of a concussion, and can be useful in monitoring recovery.

Personally, I believe that if there is a baseline on file, the first post-concussion test should be performed relatively soon following an injury —within a day or two is fine, whatever is convenient—provided that the athlete has been *medically* evaluated (to rule out any other, more serious injuries) and then retested no sooner than one week later. The goal, particularly for younger children, is for the athlete to be asymptomatic (that is, no longer experiencing any symptoms), and to complete at least two consecutive post-concussion tests (a few days apart) that reveal consistent and stable results before being allowed to begin the return-to-play process. The results of these two consecutive post-concussion tests would then help establish a new baseline for future use. Once the athlete has been cleared from a cognitive perspective, he or she should undergo physical exertional testing (more on that in the next chapter).

You don't want to over-test, however. Just as sending a concussed athlete back to school too soon can tax an overly tired brain, submitting a concussed athlete to repeated neurocognitive tests can tire him out, too. Sometimes, parents and athletes will push for faster and more frequent post-concussion testing in order to get back on the field sooner. But frequent testing does not promote faster healing. Concussions take time.

In cases where there is no baseline on file, the test interpreter should consult the testing norms (or percentile scores) to determine whether the athlete is functioning within the range considered normal. Serial testing will show the athlete's gradual improvement during the recovery phase. When the test scores no longer improve and appear stable, and the athlete has passed physical exertional testing and no longer reports any symptoms, then the most recent test will serve as the new baseline. Special care should be taken to determine when the athlete has reached his or her new baseline.

Some guidelines recommend sidelining injured athletes for one week *after* they have stopped displaying symptoms. But it is my professional opinion that a more cautious stance should be taken with children. For youth athletes, a better plan is to sideline the athlete from full-contact practices and games for three weeks after symptoms have subsided. Unfortunately, I have seen too many young athletes return to contact play too soon after feeling "back to normal" or symptom-free (that is, sooner than the recommended three weeks), only to sustain another concussion within a few weeks' time. (It should be noted, however, that an athlete who is asymptomatic, has strong cognitive test scores, and has passed physical exertional testing may return to supervised non-contact exercise and physical activity—where there is no concussion risk—a little sooner than three weeks.)

SPECIAL CIRCUMSTANCES: BASELINE TESTING FOR CHILDREN WITH ADHD OR LEARNING DISORDERS

Preseason or baseline concussion testing is arguably even more important for children with developmental conditions, including ADHD and other learning disorders. Because their test score profiles may vary and may differ from the norm, we need to know how a child with a developmental condition would usually function in order to make later post-concussion comparisons. In other words, if a child's attention is already below average, and there was no baseline testing performed, how would we know that a below-average score on post-concussion testing is actually normal for him? Likewise, very few published research studies have aimed to determine how children with developmental conditions perform on pre- and post-concussion testing. We do know, however, that children with developmental conditions tend to sustain concussions at higher rates than do other athletes, and tend to exhibit a slower recovery from concussion. If your child has been diagnosed with ADHD or a learning disorder, it is recommended that you consult a neuropsychologist to both administer and interpret baseline and post-concussion test results. Similarly, if you suspect that your child has an *undiagnosed* learning disorder or attention problem, you'll want to seek comprehensive testing through your school's child study team or school psychologist, or privately from a pediatric neuropsychologist.

CONCUSSION TESTING CONTROVERSY

Concussion testing is not without its critics. Neuropsychologist Christopher Randolph, PhD, a professor in the Department of Neurology at Loyola University Chicago Stritch School of Medicine, for example, has publicly questioned the validity of baseline testing, and has suggested that a high "false negative" rate renders baseline and post-concussion testing ineffective or even risky for young athletes (by incorrectly indicating that an injured athlete is ready to return to play).[18] And a study by Dr. Jacob Resch, director of the Brain Injury Laboratory at the University of Texas–Arlington indicated that IMPACT testing is not 100 percent reliable.[19] I think it's important to remember, though, that baseline testing is not perfect, nor should it be the only tool used in monitoring recovery from concussions or in making return-to-play decisions. Baseline testing is one tool of many and, despite its inherent flaws, it is valuable and generally considered preferable to no testing at all.

The availability of neurocognitive tests to the general public is also at issue. Neurocognitive tests are developed in a scientific manner. They are normed, or tested, on large groups of individuals to ensure validity and reliability, and the American Psychological Association governs the ethics and guidelines for their use. The sale of IMPACT, in particular, is restricted to clinics, schools, hospitals, and other reputable organizations, and requires purchasers to complete an online webinar training session and to review their testing protocols. IMPACT also provides a credentialing procedure, so that administrators may become Credentialed IMPACT Consultants (CICs). (Despite all this, of course, many schools and organizations purchase the test and then expect their athletic trainers or nurses, who are not trained neurocognitive specialists, to perform post-concussion diagnosis and treatment.)

Perhaps surprisingly, some "concussion" tests are now available for purchase to anyone with an Internet connection. One could argue, certainly, that providing the test to practically anyone anywhere may help serve disadvantaged or remote athletic populations without access to or funds for baseline testing. Unfortunately, providing unregulated access to neurocognitive tests jeopardizes the validity of the test itself.

If you are able to purchase a test on the open market, and your child is allowed to take that test in the comfort of his home, then there is nothing stopping your child (or any athlete) from practicing the test and learning its nuances, or from looking up or researching the answers, or from taking it repeatedly to improve his scores. Any of those actions would render the test invalid, and would prevent schools from being able to continue using the test to help students. It would be like handing out copies of the SAT to take at home. (I recently spoke with another concussion doctor, who told me that someone snapped a photo of a high school athlete who was taking the test for her friend!) To help ensure reliability and validity, baseline testing should be administered by trained professionals, and post-concussion testing should be administered or overseen by a neurocognitive specialist—preferably a neuropsychologist—and should not be available for use in the home or anywhere unsupervised.

Chapter 3 Review

- All youth athletes should undergo preseason or baseline cognitive testing to help facilitate return-to-play decisions if they sustain a concussion.

- Ideally, baseline testing should be performed in a quiet, controlled environment.

- Baseline tests should be reviewed for accuracy and validity.

- For additional information about neuropsychological baseline testing, including how to find a concussion testing site in your area, see page 69.

IDENTIFYING AND TREATING
YOUTH CONCUSSION
An Eight-Step Plan to Get Back in the Game

Here's the good news: a growing number of colleges and high schools across the country have finally started taking concussion prevention and management seriously. By educating athletes on the signs and symptoms of concussion, requiring baseline and post-concussion neurocognitive testing, and—most important—removing young athletes from play immediately following a brain injury (even a suspected one), we're making great strides in protecting the safety of our children, and ensuring that they will have long, happy, and healthy athletic careers. There's even a nationwide legislative movement afoot to require *all* schools and athletic programs to establish formal concussion-management programs.

Now, here's the bad news: the majority of American middle schools and elementary schools, as well as most community and recreation-based sports leagues, do not have any kind of program in place to identify, prevent, or manage concussions. As most parents know, rarely will you find an athletic trainer or other health care professional at a soccer practice for six-year-olds, or on the sidelines at a peewee football game. Rarely have youth sports coaches been educated about the dangers of a brain injury, or even shown what to look for. That means that millions and millions of young children are not only at greater risk of sustaining a concussion, but are less likely to receive the proper care and medical attention when they do get injured. Parents and coaches are often forced to navigate the confusing world of concussion aftercare alone, without any sort of guidance about where to go, what to do, who to consult, or how to help their child on the road to recovery.

This chapter outlines a detailed eight-step plan to help athletes, parents, and coaches determine *exactly* what to do if they suspect that a child has sustained a concussion. I'll also discuss alternative (less mainstream) therapies that have shown some anecdotal effectiveness in treating lingering symptoms and post-concussion syndrome. And I'll explain the frequent need for academic accommodations at school, and suggest ways to ensure that your injured athlete is getting the help he or she needs.

STEP 1: PRESEASON BASELINE TESTING

If your child's school or sports team already has a formalized concussion-management program in place (one that incorporates neurocognitive baseline testing), then step one is easy—your child will be tested automatically in the preseason, before she ever sets foot on the field. It's still a good idea, though, to check that your child is eligible to participate in the testing program. Some schools, for example, due to limited financial resources, may choose to test only varsity athletes, or may opt to establish a baseline only once (typically during the freshman year) without ever updating the scores. Don't just assume that your young athlete has undergone baseline testing, or that her baseline test is valid or up to date.

If there is no formalized concussion program in place, you can obtain private baseline testing from a sports concussion specialist. These are licensed health care professionals who have been trained in administering and interpreting preseason and post-concussion neurocognitive testing. Such individuals include neuropsychologists, as well as some physicians who specialize in sports concussion. A neurocognitive specialist can then store baseline data should it be needed for a post-concussion comparison in the future. To find a listing of neuropsychologists in your area, you can log on to the National Academy of Neuropsychology's website (nanonline.org). Or, to find a listing of CICS and test sites, log on to the IMPACT website (impacttest.com). Be aware that health insurance companies typically will not cover baseline testing because it is considered a "well visit," meaning there is no diagnosis or disease for which the child is receiving medical services. Be wary of organizations that allow you to take a baseline test in your home, without oversight or education from a concussion specialist.

Regardless of whether baseline testing is obtained in school or in a private clinic, be sure that your child, coaches, athletic trainers, and other school personnel have received some kind of training in concussion prevention and identification. The best way to identify a concussion is to know what to look for.

STEP 2: AWARENESS AND VIGILANCE

One of the most common questions I hear from both parents and coaches is, "How do I know if the athlete actually has a concussion?" Vigilance is key. Detecting a possible brain injury is relatively easy when there are obvious signs: if the child blacks out or can't keep his balance, for example. (And in such cases, you should seek immediate medical attention.) Otherwise, parents and coaches should be familiar with the behaviors of the youth athletes in their charge, and should become active observers at practices and games. Watch out for blindside hits and rough tackles, and keep a particular eye on athletes who have experienced a concussion in the past.

Both during and after a practice or game, be on the lookout for any changes in speech, balance, thinking, behavior, attention, or emotional response. Check for signs of confusion, headache, vision changes, dizziness, ringing in the ears, or nausea. Listen for slower-than-normal answers to any questions you ask. In my clinical experience, an athlete who says he feels "fine" or "okay" following a hard hit has not given you enough information. Look the child directly in the eyes and ask, slowly and methodically, "Do you feel *just like you normally would feel* after a game? Does anything feel different than usual?" Pointed questions such

> ## Did You Know . . . ?
>
> The sooner a concussed athlete starts a course of rest, the sooner his or her brain will heal. High school athletes who rested immediately following a concussion took an average of twenty-five days to recover, but those who did not needed twice as long—fifty days.[1]

as these may challenge the child to think more carefully about how he feels, and to describe any changes he may be experiencing. The answers to these questions can not only help you determine if an injury has occurred, but may also give you and your health care provider a better understanding of how your child *usually* feels. Sometimes, it's difficult to determine whether some "symptoms" are the result of a concussion, or may have been present anyway. For example, maybe your child usually has a headache after a practice or game because she suffers from sinus allergies triggered by playing in a springtime soccer field. Or, she may sometimes feel a little dizzy due to mild dehydration when playing outdoors in the heat of summer. Perhaps your child suffers from chronic ear infections, which can cause a ringing in the ears. Make a note of this kind of information, and be sure to share it with your child's doctor.

STEP 3: SIDELINE ASSESSMENT

If you suspect that a young athlete has suffered a concussion, a responsible adult should assess for immediate signs and symptoms by asking the athlete a series of questions to determine how oriented he is, and whether a loss of consciousness has occurred. Most often, that job falls to an athletic trainer (preferably certified). If no athletic trainer is present to administer a sideline assessment test, or if there is no formalized concussion questionnaire available for use, then a parent or coach can ask some simple orientation questions based on the easy-to-remember five *W*s: who, what, when, where, and why.

Who: Does the athlete know her own name? Does she know who you are?

What: What is the athlete feeling? Check for signs of amnesia, memory problems, headache, nausea, vomiting, visual disturbances (such as blurred vision), dizziness, fatigue, or confusion. Did the athlete black out or lose consciousness?

When: Does the athlete know the date, day, month, year, and approximate time of day?

Where: Does the athlete know where she is? Is she familiar with her surroundings?

Why: Determine if the athlete can explain why she is not feeling well, or why she is being examined. Can she recall events immediately before, during, and after the hit or collision? For example, can the athlete tell you that she was playing soccer against the Red Dragons when another player ran toward her and their heads collided?

As a parent or coach, you should also ask the athlete to perform some simple math calculations, depending on the child's age and maturity (for example, "What is 10 minus 7?" "What is 5 times 4?"). Next, you can instruct the athlete to listen to a random string of single-digit numbers (such as "9, 6, 2") and to recite the numbers back to you in order. If he is successful, ask him to repeat up to seven single-digit numbers in sequence. Take note of the athlete's responses to all these questions, and have the responses ready when you seek additional evaluation from a pediatrician, an emergency room doctor, or a neuropsychologist. Just make sure that any health care professional who examines the athlete is made aware of any preexisting attention or concentration difficulties, learning disorders, or ADHD, as these types of conditions can affect a child's ability to answer post-concussion questions.

The US Centers for Disease Control and Prevention (CDC) has developed a handy *Concussion Signs and Symptoms Checklist* that can be downloaded, in both English and Spanish, from the CDC website (www.cdc.gov/concussion) and used at the time of injury. A formalized sideline questionnaire called the Sport Concussion Assessment Tool (SCAT) is also available online in an updated version, SCAT2. You'll even find a Sports Concussion Card in Appendix C of this book, to copy and glue onto your coach's clipboard or hang on your refrigerator. But remember, no athlete with a suspected concussion should be returned to play, no matter how "well" he or she performs during a sideline assessment test. Some athletes may not demonstrate any significant symptoms until hours or days after impact.

STEP 4: MEDICAL EXAM

If you suspect that your child has sustained a concussion, seek an immediate medical exam. If a team physician isn't available, then you'll want to contact your pediatrician or primary care physician and schedule a quick visit. If your child attends a boarding school or college, then a visit to the student health center is in order. Ultimately, you can always take your child to the local ER.

At the ER, your child will undergo a neurological screening to make sure he hasn't suffered a more serious injury. An ER physician will want to rule out the possibility of a brain hemorrhage, and therefore may order a CT scan. (Because the brain is enclosed in the skull, the blood from a possible hemorrhage would also collect inside the skull, compressing the brain and causing swelling. This kind of bleeding might not produce symptoms for hours after an injury, but it can cause brain damage and even death if it's not detected in time. Brain hemorrhages certainly aren't common, but it's obviously best to rule out that possibility as soon as possible.) As long as all radiological studies are normal (which is typically the case with concussions), your child will most likely be sent home with instructions to follow until he can be examined by his primary care physician in an outpatient setting.

Following an uncomplicated concussion for which no radiological screenings were ordered, or when any radiological tests (for example, CT scans) that were ordered come back normal, it's important to follow these guidelines:

- Monitor your child closely for any change in or worsening of symptoms.

- Make sure your child gets plenty of rest and sleep, especially for the first few days following an injury. Even if your child is staying home from school, now is not the time to have him pitch in with housework, mow the lawn, or clean up his messy room.

- Allow no sports, gym, or athletic activity until your child is cleared by a licensed health care professional with expertise in sports concussion.

- Restrict visually stimulating activities such as computer or video games, Internet chatting, text messaging, and similar pursuits. Severely limit the amount of television your child watches, and restrict completely programs that are intense or visually stressful (no shoot-'em-up action hero films with lots of explosions, no scary movies). No reading.

- Avoid parties, trips, social activities, and stressful events.

- Preferably, allow your child to stay home from school for a day or two to help physical symptoms like headaches go away.

- Arrange for temporary academic accommodations, such as no tests or homework, with your child's teachers or school administrator. (We'll discuss this in more detail later in the chapter.)

- Follow up with a neuropsychologist for post-concussion treatment. This will typically require a series of visits, in which the sports concussion doctor will compare your child's post-concussion test results with baseline scores to help determine

True or False: You Shouldn't Be Allowed to Fall Asleep If You Have a Concussion

Parents often ask me if they need to prevent their child from falling asleep after a concussion, or if it's necessary to wake the concussed child periodically throughout the night. Actually, sleep does not hurt or endanger a concussed brain. In fact, your child will need plenty of sleep in order to heal the injury and restore the brain's electrochemical balance. However, waking a sleeping child periodically throughout the night has long been standard practice after a brain injury. That's because if a brain hemorrhage were to develop in the middle of the night, no one would know—it's not possible to detect a change in mental status or a loss of consciousness when a child is already sleeping. On the other hand, waking someone up every hour can promote fatigue, irritability, headache, and other symptoms that aren't concussion related. (If your child underwent a CT scan in the ER, and the results were normal, then there should be little concern about a brain hemorrhage, anyway.) But because each concussion is different and must be treated differently, it's best to ask your child's doctor for advice.

when the brain has fully recovered. Once symptoms have subsided and post-concussion test scores have improved, you can begin allowing your child to return to normal daily activities on a slow, gradual basis. But it's important not to rush this process. Allowing your child access to all the things he missed during the initial recovery period—video games, time on the computer, social outings, and so on—or sending him back to school too early could trigger a setback in symptoms.

· Seek physical exertional testing. Even if your child says he feels "normal" and his neurocognitive test scores look good, he should undergo physical exertional testing before beginning any type of exercise. This testing should preferably be performed by a certified athletic trainer, who will guide your child through a series of exercises to ensure that the symptoms of concussion don't return when the body is stressed.

· Schedule a follow-up appointment with your child's physician or pediatrician, or ask your neuropsychologist to communicate directly with that doctor. Even after the symptoms of concussion disappear and your child's neurocognitive tests improve, he may need to be *medically* cleared before returning to athletics. Ultimately, the decision to return to sports should be made using a team approach, and it's important that your child's health care professionals communicate with each other. No matter what, all return-to-play activity should be monitored by a licensed health care provider with training and expertise in sports concussion management. (Some state concussion laws may specifically dictate which *type* of health care professional may provide written clearance to return to school or organized athletics.)

STEP 5: EXPERT SKEPTICISM

It is extremely difficult for primary care physicians, pediatricians, and ER doctors to stay completely up to date in every specialized area of treatment, especially in frontier fields of medicine for which the guidelines change almost as quickly as a basketball score. Many doctors are playing catch-up in the area of youth concussion, and plenty are operating under old, outdated guidelines for care. That's why it's so important for parents to be educated about concussions in kids, and to be slightly skeptical of the health care advice and recommendations they receive. Don't be afraid to ask questions if a health care provider tells you something that you don't understand, or offers an opinion about concussion treatment that doesn't jibe with what you've heard or read. An intelligent, nonthreatening discussion provides the foundation for trust and a working alliance between doctor and patient. It also gives you an opportunity to determine if the doctor is up to date on concussion training and education. If, during your child's first medical exam, your health care provider says anything like the following, the alarm bells should go off:

· "Your child did not sustain a concussion because his CT scan was normal." Radiological scans are used to identify focal injuries in the brain, such as a skull fracture or brain bleed. Rarely will a concussion show up on a routine CT scan.

· "Your child should take a break from her sport, but she may return to all other normal activities." We know that immediate rest—both physical and mental—is key to a speedy recovery. Returning a child to school too soon, especially if she is still experiencing headaches or other symptoms, can actually prolong recovery, put the child at risk of developing post-concussion syndrome, and jeopardize her performance in school.

· "Your child should avoid sports for one week [or some other arbitrary period of time]." Because children heal differently, each at their own rate, it's impossible to determine how long a period of rest a particular child may need. There is no cookie-cutter protocol, no universal rule about when to allow your child back on the field, but one week is rarely enough time to recover. In fact, Robert Stern, PhD, who studies brains at the Center for the Study of Traumatic Encephalopathy, has noted than 85 percent of concussions take at least three weeks to resolve, and many take longer.[2] Every concussion is unique and must be treated individually.

STEP 6: POST-CONCUSSION OBSERVATION

Because we know that children tend to experience a delay in the onset of their symptoms, you'll want to monitor your child closely in the hours and days following a concussion. Some symptoms could indicate a more serious or even life-threatening injury (such as a brain hemorrhage) that may have gone unnoticed or undiagnosed. If your child exhibits any of the following symptoms, go to the hospital immediately.

· A worsening headache

· Extreme drowsiness, or cannot be awakened

· Difficulty recognizing people or places

· Uneven pupil dilation (one pupil looks larger than the other)

· Repeated vomiting

· Weakness or numbness in arms or legs

· Slurred speech

· Seizures

· Unusual behavior, such as increased confusion or irritability

· Difficulty maintaining balance

· Loss of consciousness

STEP 7: FOLLOWING DOCTOR'S ORDERS

It is of paramount importance that children (and their parents) abide by all post-concussion medical instructions. Failure to do so can prolong the recovery process, and could trigger a case of PCS, in which symptoms continue for anywhere from one to three months or longer following injury. Following doctor's orders, however, isn't always as easy as it sounds. At first, your child might celebrate the idea of missing a few days of school, or of postponing homework assignments and tests. But it won't take long for reality to set in: your child won't be able to play sports until he or she is medically cleared, which could take weeks.

Rest, with reduced physical and mental exertion, means no working out, no physical exercise, no attendance at practice, no text messaging, no Xbox or PlayStation or computer games, no Facebook, no trips to the mall, and no social outings or sleepovers. Those kinds of restrictions may seem like cruel punishment to a child, or like social suicide to a teenager. It's not uncommon for a concussed athlete to become distraught at such a situation. Add to that the irritability and emotional symptoms that often go hand in hand with a brain injury, and you may be looking at a rough couple of weeks. Perhaps that's why some parents attempt to negotiate the terms of post-concussion recovery with their health care provider. The following are all excuses I've heard from parents who want their children back on the field as soon as possible.

- "The college scouts will be here next week. She has to play to be seen."

- "The playoffs are this weekend, and my son is the best athlete on the team."

- "My daughter is traveling to South America with her church youth group to build homes for the poor."

The excuses go on and on. In these cases, I often find it helpful to remind the athlete and her parents of the alternative to compliance with mental rest and recovery. If she doesn't take a few days off to rest now, she may wind up missing even more practices and games, may have lingering headaches or other physical symptoms, may develop difficulty concentrating in class and have trouble performing well in school, and could be placing herself at risk for a more serious injury, such as second impact syndrome.

STEP 8: MANAGING PERSISTENT SYMPTOMS WITH ADVANCED MEDICAL CONSULTATIONS AND ALTERNATIVE THERAPIES

Currently, there is no clear, scientifically proven "cure" for concussion, other than rest and removal from mental and physical exertion. Allowing the brain time to heal itself, as well as to rebalance its electrochemical environment, is the best and most important step one can take on the road to recovery. And in most cases—when the athlete rests appropriately

Case Study No. 2

PATIENT: Stephanie; eighteen-year-old female

PREFERRED SPORT(S): Ice hockey (school and received private coaching); softball (school and private youth league); golf

FIRST APPOINTMENT WITH DR. MOSER: June 2010 (age sixteen)

TYPE OF AND DATE(S) OF INJURY:

Concussion 1: Age eight. Stephanie was ice skating at a local rink when an older boy tripped and fell on her. *Immediate symptoms*: Double vision and tingling in the extremities, which lasted through the night. Stephanie's mother took her to the pediatrician the following day. Both the CT scan and MRI results were negative (as is usually the case with concussion). Stephanie recovered smoothly and returned to school after a week spent resting at home.

Concussion 2: Age fifteen. During a school softball game, Stephanie collided with her third-base player while attempting to catch a pop fly. *Immediate symptoms*: Headache, feeling foggy. Stephanie was granted several weeks of academic accommodations by the health center at her boarding school, and was monitored by a school nurse certified in ImPACT neurocognitive testing. No other outside medical supervision.

Concussion 3: Age sixteen. The severity of Stephanie's third concussion—the one her family calls "the big one"—was likely the result of several (undiagnosed and undetected) subconcussive blows sustained over the course of one week. Stephanie, a talented ice hockey goalie, had two private coaching sessions during a February weekend. Though she deflected several pucks with her head, all seemed fine. A few days later, her regular coach also chose to spend some one-on-one practice time with her. Stephanie doesn't remember any specific save as painful or problematic, but by Thursday she was feeling out of sorts and suffering from a headache and flu-like aches and pains. On Friday, still feeling poorly, Stephanie asked her coach if she could sit out that evening's game. But when he pressured her to "suck it up and play," she did. She skated out on the ice to warm up and was accidentally whacked in the head by a teammate's hockey stick. *Immediate symptoms*: Headache, confusion, fogginess, nausea, balance difficulties, but no loss of consciousness.

Stephanie was sent to the health center for an immediate examination, and her mom drove to the boarding school to spend the weekend with her daughter. The following Monday, Stephanie was examined by the school's concussion specialist, who recommended sending her home on a temporary medical leave. But with only ten days before winter exams, Stephanie—a very conscientious student—was adamant about finishing the term. Her mother allowed her to stay, largely because she didn't realize that mental and cognitive stress could make the condition worse. When Stephanie finally came home for winter break, her condition had dramatically declined— she was sensitive to light, noise, and taste; irritable; nauseous; had difficulty concentrating; and had trouble sleeping. Her mother made an appointment with a medical doctor at a local sports medicine clinic.

INITIAL EXAM: By the time Stephanie came to see me, roughly four months after her third concussion, she was still very much in the fog of post-concussion syndrome. (An unfortunate series of accidental slips, falls, and a minor car accident between February and June may have further slowed her recovery.) Stephanie had already started working with a medical doctor at a noted sports medicine clinic, but she needed a neuropsychologist who could manage her cognitive improvement over time. Even though Stephanie had been given a preseason baseline test at her school, her Impulse Control score was greater than 30—a sign of invalidity, rendering the test results questionable at best. From a cognitive recovery perspective, then, we had to start from scratch.

RECOVERY PLAN: Immediate and extensive mental and cognitive rest: no computer, no texting, no reading, no chores, no exercise, no socializing. Lots of extra sleep. Toward the end of her recovery period, an orthopedist on Stephanie's

(continued)

(continued)

concussion-management team prescribed Amantadine, a drug used to treat Parkinson's disease that has been shown to aid in recovery from brain injuries. Stephanie also tried some alternative therapies, including craniosacral therapy, chiropractic neurology, and vestibular therapy (to "reset" her balance), all of which proved helpful. Stephanie's neurocognitive test scores also improved . . . *slowly* (probably due to her history of multiple concussion). Ultimately, Stephanie spent nearly a year under medical supervision without being cleared to return to sports.

ACADEMIC ACCOMMODATIONS: In many ways, Stephanie's school was relatively concussion savvy—every student athlete received a baseline neurocognitive test as a matter of policy (though we now know that Stephanie's test was not examined for validity). Also, Stephanie was granted academic accommodations: for example, rather than force her to take final exams at the end of winter term, her school allowed her to skip them completely, and posted her grades as they stood. On the other hand, Stephanie's case illustrates the difficulties of trying to coordinate teachers and administrators around a particular student's temporary needs, and shows how hard it can be to maintain one's academic standing while recovering from concussion. For example, Stephanie was made to take a particular proficiency exam because the proctor never got word that Stephanie was to be excused. (In her post-concussion fog, Stephanie failed to object.) She also chose to sit for a nationwide standardized test in the hope of earning scholarship money based on her scores. All of these sessions of intense cognitive engagement most likely contributed to the severity of her post-concussion decline.

NOTES: Today, Stephanie is symptom-free and has resumed a successful academic career. But her case demonstrates the potential severity of PCS, the effect of cognitive engagement on recovery, as well as the importance of a great mother-advocate. (Stephanie's mom educated herself about concussion, effectively pursued alternative therapies for her daughter, and now publicly advocates for greater concussion awareness and education.) After dealing with PCS for nearly a year, Stephanie had to make the difficult decision to end her participation in contact sports; returning to softball or ice hockey would just be too risky. But because Stephanie has so many other areas of interest, she has adapted incredibly well. These days, Stephanie acts as a student-coach for the hockey team (a great way to stay involved in one of her favorite sports), and has taken up golf.

NOTES FROM STEPHANIE'S MOM: "What I realized during the year my daughter suffered from PCS is that you really have to be an advocate for your own child; because even though Stephanie's school is reasonably concussion conscious, the management of her treatment was not as thorough as it might have been. Schools' academic offices often are not yet prepared to appropriately deal with these types of injuries, and many teachers don't yet understand the complex nature of post-concussion symptoms. There were times during Stephanie's recovery that her brain would just stop processing information—she could look at a page of words and fail to get any meaning out of a sentence. How do you explain that to a teacher who doesn't understand concussion?

"For my part, I tried to help Stephanie with her cognitive recovery at home. Once she'd completed her initial period of mental and physical rest, we looked for simple things she could do around the house. Gardening was an excellent non-strenuous activity, and books on tape required less cognitive engagement than reading. A word of warning, though: activities like organizing or de-cluttering should probably be avoided when your child is recovering from concussion. I had Stephanie help me sort some paperwork, but all that focused decision making seemed to set her back a good week's worth of progress. A concussed child needs just as much mental rest as physical rest."

and complies with doctor's orders—an uncomplicated concussion will fully resolve itself within a few weeks' time.

Sometimes, however, concussion symptoms linger. Persistent, chronic symptoms or PCS might be triggered by having returned to play too soon or having failed to comply with prescribed mental or physical rest; might be the result of multiple concussions (recovery can take significantly longer if the athlete has been concussed before); or might be related to some other extenuating circumstance or factor, such as a learning disorder or physical condition. As the science of concussion prevention and management has progressed over the years, some alternative therapies have gained traction as possibly beneficial. The following types of advanced medical consultations and alternative therapies may be helpful if your child is suffering from the prolonged effects of a concussive blow.

Advanced Medical Consultations

Neurological consultation. When headaches or other symptoms persist, a neurological consultation may be in order. A neurologist is a physician who specializes in the central nervous system, including the brain, nerves, and spinal cord. He or she can help rule out complicating factors that may have been missed, or that may not be related to the concussive injury itself. A neurologist may choose to order a series of tests, including MRI, which examines the functioning of the brain, or EEG, to check for any irregularity in brain waves or possible seizure activity. Neurologists, in particular, are trained in treating headaches through medical/pharmacological intervention.

Biofeedback consultation. Another treatment that's been proven effective for persistent headaches and migraines is biofeedback, in which a specialist uses a biofeedback machine and skin sensors to receive instant data about the body's physical state, including skin temperature, muscle tension, and pulse rate. Then the specialist works with the patient to relax, control, and ultimately change these states. By learning to relax, patients can reduce any tension that may be contributing to headaches or other symptoms. There are no needles or invasive devices involved in biofeedback, though it usually requires multiple sessions per week over a period of several weeks.

Pharmacologic consultation. Generally speaking, pharmacologic therapies (that is, prescription medications) are used to treat certain *symptoms* of concussion—such as headaches, sleep disturbances, or emotional problems—rather than the actual concussion itself. In fact, there is no type of medication that can actually cure a brain injury. With children, it's often best to avoid unnecessary pharmacologic intervention whenever possible, although some concussions are severe and persistent enough to necessitate some kind of drug therapy.

Psychotropic medications (such as antidepressants and anxiolytics) are sometimes prescribed to treat symptoms of depression and anxiety that may arise from a brain injury, particularly in cases where an athlete has been concussed multiple times and should no longer engage in any kind of organized athletics (a traumatic, emotional situation, to be sure). Because concussions alter the brain chemistry, symptoms such as irritability, anger, sadness, tearfulness, moodiness, depression, and anxiety are not uncommon. You may want to consider making an appointment for your child to see a psychiatrist (one who understands concussions) if he or she is experiencing emotional or behavioral problems.

Neuro-ophthalmological consultation. Patients with persistent visual difficulties may want to consult a neuro-ophthalmologist, a physician who specializes in the part of the nervous system that governs vision and the functions of the eye.

Counseling and psychotherapy consultation. Adjusting to the chronic nature of PCS, and the ways it may alter lifestyle and everyday functioning, is not easy. Talking to a specialist can help ease some of the stress and pressure, and can help the athlete find better ways to compensate for any difficulties and changes. Finding a counselor or psychotherapist who understands mild brain injury is key. Also, some concussion specialists offer support groups for kids who are coping with PCS and managing the demands of school.

Novel or Alternative Therapies

The following types of therapies are still in the research stage.

Neurofeedback. Similar to biofeedback, neurofeedback is a way to monitor the brain's electrical activity with the use of noninvasive sensors. The patient is taught to alter her brain's response to certain stimuli through practice and repetition in order to control and reduce symptoms of concussion as well as to improve attention and concentration. (Basically, the idea is to normalize your brain wave patterns.) Neurofeedback is also sometimes used in the treatment of depression, anxiety, and ADHD. Sessions tend to be costly, however, and often are not covered by insurance.

Epsom salt footbaths. Magnesium is a vital element in myriad brain and bodily functions, yet most people in the United States probably aren't getting enough. Mild magnesium deficiency has been linked to everything from ADHD, asthma, and migraine headaches to neurological symptoms such as tremors or muscle spasms (though only in very severe cases). Supplemental magnesium, on the other hand, has been used to help treat all these conditions, as well as to promote recovery from severe brain injuries. Magnesium is also one of two main elements that make up Epsom salt, the type of salt crystals that people have been adding to their bath water for years, to soften skin and relieve muscle tension. (The other element, by the way, is sulfate. Interestingly, some evidence suggests that sulfate deficiency may play a role in autism.)

When you soak your feet in an Epsom salt bath, magnesium and sulfate are absorbed by your body through the skin. Although the evidence is very, very preliminary, some experts believe that this supplemental magnesium may help alleviate some symptoms of concussion and promote recovery from brain injury. Epsom salts are available in any grocery or health food store, and are generally considered safe to use (though you should always speak to a doctor before starting any kind of supplement program).

Docosahexaenoic acid (DHA). DHA is a type of omega-3 fatty acid and a building block of brain tissue. DHA can be found in fish, especially tuna, cod, and Atlantic salmon, and can be derived from certain types of algae and taken in supplement form. A growing number of studies suggest that a diet high in DHA can aid in brain development. One study in particular found that, within the first six months of life, babies born to mothers with higher levels of DHA in their blood were developmentally "two months ahead" of babies born to mothers with lower levels of DHA; this is one reason that some infant formulas and baby foods are now DHA-fortified.[3] More recent research has suggested that DHA may also aid in the treatment of and recovery from concussion. The University of Georgia, for example, has already added the use of algal DHA supplements (3 grams daily for thirty days, or until the athlete is asymptomatic) to its official post-concussion policy for all athletes.[4, 5] The American military, meanwhile, is considering including DHA supplements in the rations of all active-duty service members, in part to speed recovery from possible brain injuries.[6]

Craniosacral therapy. Inside your skull, your brain is floating around in a cushion of protective cerebrospinal fluid. That fluid also lubricates the spine; it flows from your brain all the way down to your sacrum, which is the main bone at the base of the spine, right above the tailbone. The craniosacral system, as it's called, includes this cerebrospinal fluid as well as bones and membranes, and it influences the functioning and health of the central nervous system (that is, your brain and spinal cord).

Craniosacral therapy is a type of alternative holistic therapy, generally practiced by osteopaths, massage therapists, or chiropractors. It uses very light touch (considerably lighter than a massage) to monitor the craniosacral system and the flow of cerebrospinal fluid, to alleviate tension, to increase blood flow to the brain, and to relax and "balance" the body. It's most often used to alleviate migraines, neck and back pain and other chronic pain conditions, and orthopedic problems, as well as conditions such as ADHD and autism. Although research is lacking on the use of craniosacral therapy in the recovery from mild traumatic brain injury (mTBI), I have had a few parents tell me that it was helpful for their children.

Acupuncture. Acupuncture is an ancient Chinese alternative therapy that involves inserting tiny needles into various pressure points on the body (often on the face and ears). It has been used to relieve pain, treat infertility, prevent disease, and improve overall health, but it has more recently gained popularity as a treatment for the symptoms of concussion. Several branches of the military, for example, including the US Navy and Marine Corps, have begun to embrace the use of acupuncture—or "battlefield acupuncture," as they call it—in the treatment of concussed military personnel.[7]

Vestibular rehabilitation therapy (VRT). The vestibular system, located in the inner ear, controls your body's equilibrium and balance. Understandably, then, problems with the vestibular system can cause dizziness, vertigo, Ménière's disease (characterized by periodic ringing in the ears, progressive hearing loss, episodes of vertigo, and balance difficulties), and other symptoms. For some people, the brain may automatically compensate for a vestibular problem on its own, and any symptoms will subside after a few weeks' time. For others, VRT may be necessary.

VRT is a type of physical therapy that incorporates head, body, and eye exercises in order to "reset" the brain to compensate for balance issues. Recent research has indicated that VRT may also help alleviate symptoms such as dizziness and headache in athletes with post-concussion syndrome, even if the patient doesn't seem to have any actual balance difficulties.

Off-label pharmaceuticals. Amantadine (brand names Symadine and Symmetrel) is a type of prescription medication that's generally used for the treatment of Parkinson's disease, though some studies have shown that it may also aid in the recovery from concussion. Personally, I've seen a number of patients with PCS whose neurologists placed them on Amantadine; it seemed to jump-start the ending of their symptoms, particularly the mental fogginess.

Researchers are also looking into the possibility that Posiphen, an experimental Alzheimer's drug, may have some bearing on recovery from mild traumatic brain injury (MTBI).

It's important to point out that most of these therapies are still in experimental, preliminary stages, and have not yet been scientifically proven to have an effect on the treatment of concussion. Novel and alternative therapies should be tried only at the advice of and under the supervision of a trained, licensed health care professional. Don't hesitate to speak to your doctor if your child is suffering from prolonged or lingering symptoms of concussion.

ACADEMIC ACCOMMODATIONS

For many children—particularly those who are still experiencing physical symptoms of concussion, including headaches or dizziness, several days after the initial injury—returning to school will be incredibly challenging. Even students whose physical symptoms have subsided may still have difficulty staying focused in the classroom or keeping pace with their regular schoolwork. Concussions, remember, are a cognitive injury, so it's not uncommon for an injured athlete's grades to slip or for his behavior to change in the weeks and months ahead. In fact, in a survey of concussed children and their parents, researchers at the Children's National Medical Center in Washington, DC, found that 65 percent of concussed athletes aged ten to eighteen had trouble paying attention in class, 61 percent felt that their homework assignments took too long to complete, and 55 percent had difficulty studying for tests and quizzes in the sixty days following injury.[8] The best way to ease your child's transition back to school is to arrange for temporary academic accommodations— such as extended time for homework and tests, and no gym class or recess play—for a period of days, weeks, or even longer in more severe cases.

In my experience, most schools are supportive when it comes to providing these types of temporary academic accommodations. If your child's school has no written concussion policy or procedure to support recovery, however, you may need to be more proactive. Talk to your child's teachers, guidance counselor, athletic trainer, and coaches. Make sure that everyone is aware of your child's injury and symptoms. Explain any difficulties your child has in maintaining focus and concentration, as well as any physical problems (such as headache, fatigue, or dizziness) that may affect his performance in class. Providing this kind of information to teachers and administrators will not only help ensure that your child gets the kind of educational support he needs, but will also aid in the monitoring of his physical recovery. By bringing everyone up to speed on your child's condition, teachers and administrators will know what to watch for, and will be better able to report to you, directly and quickly, any change in or worsening of symptoms.

But remember, the best way to determine the kinds of academic accommodations that might be necessary is to consult with your child's neuropsychologist or sports concussion specialist. These doctors are trained in evaluating neurocognitive post-concussion testing. Additionally, they are sensitive to the emotional component of recovery from concussion (neuropsychologists, in particular, understand the irritability and frustration that often come with a brain injury). They can also custom tailor an academic plan for your child, and they can communicate their recommendations directly to school officials, as well as provide any medical documentation that might be necessary in securing those academic accommodations.

Here are some of the most common types of academic accommodations available for concussed children with lingering symptoms:

· The athlete may require a few days, or in more severe cases, even a few weeks off from school—with no homework or assignments—until the bulk of the headaches and other physical symptoms subside. It's not actually necessary for a concussed athlete to stay in bed all day, but she should get plenty of sleep, and during this time you should continue to restrict her mental and physical exertion (including limiting access to video games, computer, and visually stimulating television shows).

· Depending on how the athlete feels after a few additional days of rest, he may need to return to school on a half-day or alternating-day basis, with allotted breaks and time to rest (perhaps visiting the nurse or a quiet study hall), before slowly transitioning back to full days. During this time, and until he is medically cleared by a licensed health care professional, he should be excused from gym class and all other forms of exercise. He may also need to have some tests postponed, any computer use in the classroom restricted, and homework assignments excused, or may need additional time for tests and assignments. In the survey I mentioned earlier, from the National Children's Medical Center in Washington, DC, a majority of respondents (52.8 percent) indicated that the specific academic accommodation that was most helpful or most needed was additional time to complete assignments and tests, followed by a reduction of homework, and rest breaks throughout the school day. Preferential seating in class (in the front, nearest the teacher, and away from doors and windows) may also help your child stay focused and attentive.

· Putting too much pressure on your child to make up all of her missed assignments immediately when she returns to school is not only stressful, it's not really fair. After all, if we understand that a concussed athlete may have difficulty keeping up with a regular course load, how could we expect her to complete all the makeup work simultaneously? So, devise a plan for her to make up missed assignments. Work with her teachers and guidance counselor to determine which of the assignments are absolutely essential to complete, and which might be excused. (If a child has already mastered a specific concept, there probably isn't a need for her to make up four additional assignments on that same concept.) Consider asking that some exams be completed orally, rather than on paper. If your child has fallen considerably behind, you might want to arrange for private tutoring to complete assignments, or for makeup classes to be held during vacation.

· Remember that each concussion is unique, and it's impossible to predict the potential need for academic accommodations at the time of injury. Therefore, each recovery plan should be considered unique and flexible, and requires a tailored return-to-school and return-to-play process. Likewise, your child's performance in each individual school subject may differ slightly. For example, research studies show that math class tends to trigger the most problems for concussed children, and is the subject for which parents and their children most often report dropping grades or grades that are at risk of dropping. If that's the case for your child, then he may need a longer period of academic accommodation (for example, more time allotted for tests and quizzes, or homework reduction) for math class than, say, language arts.[8]

In more extreme, chronic cases, when concussion symptoms linger for weeks on end, or when symptoms are severe enough that they are intolerable or interfere with learning and school performance, more elaborate academic accommodations may need to be put in place. These options include the following:

> *504 plan or Individualized Education Program (IEP).* Schools are legally required to identify and accommodate children with disabilities, physical handicaps, diseases, and injuries to ensure that they get the same quality education as every other child. This is often accomplished by creating a 504 plan or an IEP; both are types of written documents that clearly spell out any special academic accommodations needed for a particular student. Because both 504 plans and IEPs are legal documents, they each require a series of official steps (read: *each carries a fair amount of bureaucratic red tape*). You may have to formally request a 504 plan or an IEP in writing to initiate the process, and your doctor may have to submit some necessary paperwork to document your child's need for additional accommodations.

> *Temporary home schooling.* Home schooling reduces the amount of time each day that is devoted to academics and provides an individualized one-to-one teaching environment. One or two teachers may be assigned to meet with the student for a few hours each day, or a few times each week. Very often, students find that they can cover more academic material in less time and more efficiently, leaving greater time for resting the brain. This kind of home schooling may require a 504 plan.

Medical leave of absence. In the worst-case scenario, a medical leave of absence may be necessary so that the concussed brain can undergo a period of comprehensive, extended rest. In some cases, students may be able to make up some of the school time missed over a summer break. In other cases, students may actually need to repeat a grade or semester.

Chapter 4 Review

· The best way to identify a concussion is to know what to look for. Educate yourself on the signs and symptoms of brain injury, and observe your child closely during and after practices and games for signs of concussion and changes in behavior. Be vigilant.

· If your child sustains a concussion, you should follow your concussion doctor's orders. The most important step in a speedy recovery is getting plenty of mental and physical rest. That means no exercise, no sports, no reading (books, magazines, homework), no computer, and no video games. Failure to rest properly can make the concussion worse and prolong the recovery process.

· Monitor your child closely in the hours and days following a concussive injury. A rapid decline in his condition, or the appearance of symptoms such as extreme drowsiness, repeated vomiting, or a worsening headache are all signs that he should be taken to a hospital immediately.

· Be an advocate for your child. Don't be afraid to request or arrange for academic accommodations at her school right away, especially if she is struggling with lingering symptoms, or to discuss alternative therapies or other medical consultations with her doctor.

WHEN IN DOUBT, SIT THEM OUT
Making Responsible Return-to-Play Decisions

In early October 2005, nineteen-year-old sophomore Preston Plevretes, a lineman on the LaSalle University football team, head-butted another player during an afternoon practice. Four days later, still suffering from debilitating headaches and vision problems, he removed himself from a game against Marist University and discussed his symptoms with his athletic trainer. He was later examined by a nurse at the university health center, and underwent a CT scan and eye exam at the local emergency room, but the tests proved unremarkable. By mid-October, Plevretes was cleared to return to play. But he didn't tell his doctors that he was still suffering from headaches; only a few of his teammates had any idea.[1]

On November 4, the LaSalle football team traveled to Pittsburgh to battle it out against Duquesne University. With only minutes remaining in the fourth quarter, Plevretes collided with an opposing player head-on and collapsed on the field. In a matter of seconds, Plevretes had developed a life-threatening blood clot, which put immense pressure on his rapidly swelling brain: he suffered three strokes and lapsed into a coma en route to Mercy Hospital, located just a few blocks away from Duquesne's Rooney Field. By the time Plevretes was wheeled into the operating room, neurosurgeon Eric Altschuler thought the patient looked more like a high-speed car crash victim than a football player. "We were all quite surprised at how badly he was hurt and how quickly he went downhill," Altschuler later told the *Pittsburgh Post-Gazette*. "We couldn't believe this was from a football injury. Clearly, the worst brain injury we've seen from football."[1]

Today, after multiple surgeries, stem-cell transplants, and years of aggressive therapies, Plevretes remains wheelchair-bound, has significant speech and memory problems, and needs an aid to assist him. In a video filmed for ESPN.com, Plevretes struggles to say, "I could have sat out a season. But now I will sit out for the rest of my life."[2] His injury resulted in a $7.5 million legal settlement from LaSalle University and made waves in the world of college athletics.

Although cases of second impact syndrome are mercifully infrequent, the consequences are obviously catastrophic, and often fatal. That's why it's simply not possible to overstate the dangers of sending a concussed athlete back on the field too soon. In the days and weeks following a concussive blow, the brain is incredibly vulnerable to a second injury. More than anything else, concussions need time to heal.

Despite everything we've learned about concussion recovery in the past few years, however, research tells us that many—if not most—pediatric, family practice, and ER doctors and nurses are not up to date on the latest return-to-play guidelines; and that the care concussed children receive, particularly in hospitals, really hasn't improved all that much over time. A 1995 study of discharge instructions for youth athletes at Children's Hospital of Alabama, for example, revealed that only ten of thirty-three concussed youth athletes received what would be considered "appropriate" aftercare instructions. Of the remaining patients, twenty didn't receive any kind of instruction or documentation about when it would be safe to return to play, and three patients were actually told to return to sports too soon.[3]

By 2001, doctors and nurses weren't faring much better. Researchers asked a group of pediatric, family practice, and ER physicians, as well as pediatric and family nurse practitioners in the Rochester, New York, area to determine when an athlete should be instructed to return to sports based on three hypothetical concussion scenarios (respondents were instructed to select one of four possible multiple-choice answers). Only

7.6 percent of those surveyed responded correctly to the first scenario, which described a "mild" concussion with no loss of consciousness.[4] A more recent 2008 study further confirmed that youth athletes with a sports-related concussion receive inconsistent medical care, at best.[5]

Through legislative efforts and federally funded concussion-management programs, brain injury advocates hope to standardize the care our children receive in hospitals and doctors' offices around the country. In the meantime, it's up to parents to ensure the safety of their children's brains. The goal of this chapter is to eliminate the chance of returning a youth athlete to play too soon, and to provide parents with a clear understanding of the steps to follow before their concussed athlete steps back onto the field.

HOW DO I KNOW WHEN IT'S SAFE?
STEP-BY-STEP RETURN-TO-PLAY GUIDELINES

The single most important rule of thumb to follow after a concussion is this: No child should *ever* be returned to play if he or she is experiencing symptoms. It doesn't matter what those symptoms are, how many symptoms the child has, or how severe those symptoms seem to be; the presence of any symptom indicates that the child is still in recovery, and that returning to play would be incredibly dangerous. Yet many athletes—particularly children—are not always willing or able to admit to or describe their symptoms. And sometimes they don't even know what the symptoms of concussion are. It's not safe, then, to rely solely on the athlete to tell you when he or she is feeling better. Instead, you'll want to follow these guidelines before allowing a concussed athlete back on the field:

> · *Schedule a medical exam.* As discussed in the previous chapter, skull fractures, brain hemorrhages, and other types of focal injuries following a concussive event are thankfully infrequent, but you'll want to make sure that your child has not sustained a more serious neurological or physical injury

> ## Did You Know . . . ?
>
> Computerized tomography (otherwise known as a CT or CAT scan) may be requested by an examining physician if you take your child to the ER. The test may be ordered either with or without *contrast*, which is a dye that is injected into the patient, travels to the brain, and provides doctors with more visual detail during the imaging process.

before you take him home. Your doctor may order a CT scan or some other form of neurological screening—depending on the type and severity of symptoms—to rule out these kinds of injuries. But even if your child's test results are "normal" or "negative," this doesn't mean that he did not sustain a concussion, nor does it mean that he's ready to return to play. Symptoms of brain injuries can show up several days after a rough tackle or a hard hit, so you'll want to monitor your child closely for any changes in his behavior or worsening of his symptoms.

· *Give the brain a chance to heal.* A brief period of comprehensive mental and physical rest is the single most important step in recovery. Make sure your child complies with all of his doctor's orders. A few days off from school may be necessary until his symptoms go away.

· *Arrange for post-concussion neurocognitive testing.* Even if your child never had preseason baseline testing performed, post-concussion testing can still prove helpful in determining when he's healed from his injury. The neuropsychologist will administer the test several times over the course of a few days or weeks (depending on the severity of the concussion) and compare your child's scores to his baseline (if one was performed), or monitor improvement and compare to normative data for your child's age (if there is no baseline). Once the athlete reaches or exceeds his baseline, he'll be able to proceed to the next step *provided he is no longer experiencing any physical, cognitive, emotional/behavioral, or sleep symptoms.* The persistence of these symptoms indicates that the athlete has not healed and is not ready to return to sports, regardless of the results of post-concussion testing.

· *Undergo physical exertional testing and gradual reconditioning.* Once the athlete's symptoms have subsided and his neurocognitive tests have returned to baseline or better, he should undergo physical exertional testing to make sure that his symptoms don't return when the body is stressed. Typically, this kind of exertion testing should be performed by a certified athletic trainer, a sports medicine physician, or some other trained health care provider, who will progressively guide the athlete through activities such as running or stationary cycling, gradually increasing the duration of exercise over time. If at any time during physical exertional testing the athlete's symptoms reappear, he should return to mental and physical rest for a day or two more before trying again.

In some cases, an athletic trainer might also use the Balance Error Scoring System, or BESS testing, which assesses the athlete's balance and equilibrium through three twenty-second tests (standing on one foot, standing on a medium-density piece of foam, and so on). BESS testing is scored subjectively by the test administrator, meaning that the scoring isn't perfect, and it's subject to human error. While researchers are attempting to computerize the scoring process to eliminate the chance for error, BESS testing is still considered a useful tool by concussion specialists.

Once your child has passed physical exertional testing, he still won't be ready to return to full-contact practice or regular game play right away. The body and the brain both need time to adjust to being active again, especially if your child has been resting for several weeks. By slowly working his way up a "ladder" of physical activity, he can rebuild his coordination and confidence, and lessen the chance that any post-concussion symptoms will return.

In November 2008, a group of doctors met in Zurich, Switzerland, for the third annual Conference on Concussion in Sport to address concussion identification, treatment, and return-to-play guidelines. The official position paper from the conference outlines the following step-by-step process to ensure that an athlete isn't moving too quickly or pushing her body too hard.[6] As long as your child remains asymptomatic at each progressive stage of physical activity—that is, as long as her symptoms don't return—then she can move from one step to the next on a day-by-day basis. (So each step should take a minimum of twenty-four hours, or about one week total to complete.) But if any symptoms return, your child should drop back down a level, rest for a period of twenty-four hours, and try again to proceed to the next step. It's also important to note that no athlete should proceed to Steps 5 or 6, or return to any full-contact practices or games, without first receiving written medical clearance from a licensed health care professional.

Step 1. *No physical activity.* The athlete should be on complete mental and physical rest following a concussion until she is no longer exhibiting any symptoms.

Step 2. *Light aerobic exercise.* Once medically cleared to start physical exertion, the athlete can engage in light, low-impact exercise, such as running, swimming, or stationary cycling. Experts recommend that the athlete keep the intensity at or below 70 percent of maximum target heart rate and avoid resistance training (or weight training) at this stage. Though an athletic trainer or physician can help determine your child's target heart rate, the general idea here is to take it easy. Pushing oneself too hard, too fast, can trigger a recurrence of physical symptoms, and can set the athlete back in her recovery.

Step 3. *Sport-specific exercise.* This might entail running drills for a soccer player, skating drills in ice hockey, or shooting drills on the basketball court. The athlete should still avoid any risk of head impact at this stage, so no pads or tackling in football, no heading the ball in soccer, and so on.

Step 4. *Non-contact training drills.* The athlete may progress to more complicated training drills, but should still avoid physical contact; that might entail passing drills for a football or ice hockey player. The athlete may begin progressive resistance or weight training.

Step 5. *Full-contact practice.* The athlete can return to all normal training activities.

Step 6. *Normal game play.* The athlete has reached full return-to-play status.

· *Receive medical clearance from a physician or licensed health care professional with expertise in concussion management.* After the athlete's physical and cognitive symptoms have subsided, his neurocognitive tests have returned to baseline or better, and he undergoes physical exertional testing and graduated, non-contact exercise without a recurrence of symptoms, you should obtain formal, medical clearance to return to sports from a doctor who specializes in concussion management. Often, this will be a neuropsychologist or sports medicine physician with concussion training. Some state laws actually dictate who should provide the final clearance for return to school sports, so become familiar with any concussion laws in your state (you can read more about these in Chapter 7). In any case, your child's regular physician or pediatrician will want to know the results of the neurocognitive and physical exertional testing, and should consult with the concussion specialists treating your child.

As noted in Chapter 4, it is my recommendation that concussed youth athletes not return to contact risk for at least three weeks after all symptoms have subsided. Although that may sound like an excessively long break, a recent study showed that cerebral blood flow in youth may remain suppressed even 30 days after a concussion.[7] In my experience, by the time an athlete has completed an initial course of rest, submitted to post-concussion testing, and passed physical exertional testing and a graduated return to exercise, three weeks or so have already passed anyway. Better not to rush the recovery process; returning to sports too soon only sets the athlete up for further, potentially devastating injuries.

WHY HELMETS CAN'T PREVENT CONCUSSIONS

Lots of parents believe they can protect their children from brain injuries just by purchasing the newest, most expensive sporting equipment. But the truth is that no helmet can fully prevent concussion. In fact, football helmets, for example, are designed primarily to prevent skull fractures and scalp lacerations; that's the only sort of certification required by the National Operating Committee on Standards for Athletic Equipment (NOCSAE), a privately funded group that oversees the safety of athletic equipment in the United States. NOCSAE's current method of *drop-testing*, wherein helmets are literally dropped from varying heights and tested to determine how well they absorb and diffuse the resulting force, has been in place since 1973 (not exactly a new, evolving standard of safety, as many critics often point out).[8]

It's not that athletic equipment companies don't *want* to manufacture a helmet that prevents brain injuries. The problem is that we can't quite figure out how to do it. Remember, concussions aren't always caused by a blow to the head; a tackle to the chest or a collision with another player can produce enough whiplash-like force to slam the brain against the interior of the skull. Some scientists and researchers have therefore theorized that the mechanism of concussion is so complex that helmets will never be able to prevent concussion any more than they already do. As

> ### Did You Know . . . ?
>
> USA Hockey players and athletes governed by the National Federation of State High School Associations (NFHS) are all required to wear hockey headgear that has been certified by the Hockey Equipment Certification Council (HECC). All helmets are drop-tested, face protectors undergo puck and face blade hits, and chin straps are tested for strength and elongation. (Non-goalie helmet certification lasts for six and one-half years, so check your child's helmet sticker. Unfortunately—and surprisingly—goalie helmets are not subjected to the same standards or testing as are non-goalie helmets, and there is no standard regarding expiration of certification: a frightening fact, considering that goalies are frequently hit with the force of a flying puck.) In contrast to youth football, youth ice hockey participation typically allows players and parents to individually choose and purchase their own helmets. Visit the HECC website (www.hecc.net) for product certification and testing of helmets, chin straps, visors, and full-face protectors.

reported by the *New York Times*, NOCSAE's technical director, David Halstead, explained this conundrum at the board's annual meeting in January 2011: "We've got a lot of information, but we don't know what to do next."[8]

This confusion is largely why NOCSAE and helmet manufacturers do not release their in-house testing data to the public at large. There is widespread belief that allowing consumers access to the data—without a proper understanding of how that data was collected or how the testing itself works—would cause people to make incorrect assumptions about the safety of a particular helmet. But this means that there is no way for a parent, coach, or athletic trainer to compare one helmet against another using some kind of independent safety rating, the way you might compare the crash-test results from, say, one mid-sized sedan to another before purchasing a vehicle.

Things get even more complicated when you consider the fact that

NOCSAE is funded largely by the industry itself, and its board includes representatives from some of the leading equipment manufacturers. This apparent conflict of interest has left some critics more than a little suspicious, and has even prompted investigations into some companies' advertising claims, as well as industry-wide testing practices, by both the US Consumer Product Safety Commission and the Federal Trade Commission.[9] It's also what prompted Stefan Duma, an engineering professor at Virginia Tech, to launch the first football helmet rating system, based on eight years of data and statistical analysis, and to share his results with the general public.[10]

According to Duma's Virginia Tech National Impact Database, released in May 2011, the following were the safest adult football helmets on the market (prices are included for comparison purposes, and are current as of this writing): the Riddell Revolution Speed ($243.99), the only helmet to receive the maximum 5-star rating; followed by the 4-star-rated helmets Schutt ION 4D ($259.95), Schutt DNA Pro+ ($169.95), Xenith X1 ($299.99), Riddell Revolution ($182.99), and Riddell Revolution IQ ($222.99). On the opposite end of the spectrum, the Dumas study found that the recently discontinued Riddell VSR-4, the most widely used helmet in the NFL during the 2010 season, as well as the helmet worn by roughly half of the Virginia Tech team and about 75,000 high school and college athletes nationwide—not to mention the company's best seller—performed comparatively poorly, earning a rating of only 1 star. (Only one of the ten helmets tested scored lower than the Riddell VSR-4: the Adams A2000 Pro Elite [$199.95] earned a rating of Not Recommended, or 0 stars.) As a result of Duma's study, Virginia Tech players formerly wearing the VSR-4 switched to the 5-star Riddell Revolution Speed helmet in the fall of 2011.

Duma has been quick to point out that there is no correlation between helmet price and performance, shattering the notion that a more expensive helmet would result in better protection from concussive blows. And he further claimed that "you can cut your risk of concussion by 55 percent by switching from the VSR-4 to the Xenith X1," in a statement to the *New York Times*.[11] Yet his research is not without limitations. First, only adult helmets intended for use by players of high school age and older were included in the study, so the results aren't applicable to youth helmets. Second, the study uses the same type of drop-testing that NOCSAE requires, so it doesn't account for concussions sustained by rotational forces (because there still isn't an approved scientific method by which to do so).

For its part, NOCSAE is doing what it can to push for newer and safer football helmets for youth athletes, in part by funding independent research on the subject, as well as by partnering with government agencies to promote greater awareness of concussion management and prevention. To further address the problem of helmet safety, US Senator Tom Udall of New Mexico and US Representative Bill Pascrell Jr. of New Jersey recently introduced an athletic equipment safety bill, which would require third-party oversight of helmet manufacturing, updated labels on helmets (including reconditioned ones), and severe penalties for helmet manufacturers that make misleading safety claims. But until such a law has been passed and significant improvements by manufacturers have been made, it's important for parents to do the following:

· *Know what kind of athletic equipment your children are using.* The vast majority of youth athletes use reconditioned helmets (that is, helmets that have been sent to a reconditioning company for inspection and recertification). Studies show that only about one of every five high school football helmets is new.[12] Though there's nothing wrong with using reconditioned equipment per se, there is some evidence to suggest that reconditioning companies don't always properly abide by NOCSAE guidelines. We also know that schools and community sports leagues with limited funding may not have their equipment reconditioned often enough (experts suggest every one to three years), or may use equipment for longer than is advisable (the National Athletic Equipment

Reconditioning Association [NAERA] no longer accepts football helmets that are more than ten years old).[13] Ask your child's coach or athletic trainer what type of equipment the team provides, and how often it is sent for recertification.

· *Educate yourself on the latest helmet technology.* Generally speaking, newer helmets incorporate newer technology and *may* lessen the risk of concussion in youth athletes. For example, the Xenith X1 helmet, which NOCSAE vice president Dr. Robert Cantu has called "the greatest advance in helmet design in the last 30 years," incorporates eighteen shock-absorbing disks rather than the more traditional foam padding.[14] (Full disclosure: Dr. Cantu is a Xenith advisor.) Other companies, including Riddell and Schutt, have also made great strides in the types of interior padding used.

· *Band together.* Perhaps the single greatest challenge to most school- and community-based athletic programs is a lack of funding. When an athletic program does not have the money to secure new or properly reconditioned equipment for its athletes, parents should be allowed to privately purchase equipment or organize fund-raisers for the purchasing of equipment. By banding together and buying in bulk, parents may be able to secure large discounts and outfit an entire team (rather than a few privileged individuals) with the best equipment available. Xenith's One Player One Helmet program, for example, allows for parents, rather than the football program itself, to help pay for helmets through tax-deductible donations.[15] In turn, the program tracks each helmet's specific maintenance history through the use of a serial number, ensuring that the component parts (interior padding, and so on) are not of indeterminate age and questionable effectiveness.

What We Know about
Mouth Guards and Concussion

Just as medical researchers and manufacturers are working to create a helmet that's truly effective at preventing concussion, the need for a safer, better-quality mouth guard has grown considerably, too. Yet research on the subject is surprisingly limited, and the results are usually inconclusive at best. Some studies, for example, indicate that mouth guards don't reduce the risk of concussion at all; some suggest that mouth guards are effective at preventing more catastrophic or severe head injuries only; and some claim that they're so often worn incorrectly (or not at all) that their potential effectiveness is rendered null and void.[16-18] Despite these findings, however, we actually *have* come a long way from the simple "boil-and-bite" moldable plastic mouth guards that are available at your local sporting goods store.

High-quality, custom-fit models are made from dental impressions of the teeth, so they typically fit better, won't wear down, won't fall out, and won't make speech or breathing difficult (all issues that might prevent a child from wearing a mouth guard as often as necessary). There is also some evidence to suggest that certain kinds of custom-fit mouth guards may be able to displace or reduce the level of g-force resulting from an impact to the jaw—this *may* lessen the likelihood that a bump to the face will produce a concussive blow. Many of the leading brands of custom-fit mouth guards provide at-home self-impression kits that you can return to the manufacturer, eliminating the need for an expensive trip to the dentist. Just remember that no mouth guard will reduce the risk of or prevent concussion completely (no matter what the packaging or advertisements claim), and even children outfitted with the best available equipment must be educated on the signs and symptoms of brain injury.

HOW MANY CONCUSSIONS ARE *TOO* MANY?
THE LONG-TERM EFFECTS OF BRAIN INJURY

It's obvious that no amount of injury is *good* for the brain. And unfortunately, there is no magic number to determine how many concussions are too many. Every child is different, and every concussion is different. However, the more concussions a child sustains, the more likely he or she is to experience cognitive, emotional, and behavioral problems later in life. In other words, the effects of multiple concussions compound over time.

For example, we already know that recently concussed child athletes perform more poorly on tests of memory, attention, and concentration than do their uninjured peers; that's why neurocognitive testing is so useful. Neuropsychologists are able to determine when an athlete has likely healed, based on the improvement in his or her post-concussion test scores. What's particularly interesting, though, is that there may not be much difference, cognitively speaking, between a child who has *recently* sustained a concussion and a child who has sustained at least two previous concussions at some point in his or her athletic career. It appears that once a child has sustained two or more concussions, his or her performance on subtle tasks of attention and processing speed may not be too different from the performance of an athlete who sustained a concussion *within the previous week.*[19]

Recent research has also shown us that children who have experienced multiple concussions at some point in their athletic careers tend to report more and worse immediate symptoms (such as loss of consciousness, amnesia, and confusion) when injured again, compared to athletes who've only had one or fewer brain injuries.[20] Children with a history of multiple concussions also report more long-lasting symptoms, take longer to recover, and tend to have lower cumulative grade point averages (GPAs).

Further complicating matters is the fact that having sustained one concussion makes an athlete four to six times more likely to sustain another. In one study of high school and college football players, athletes who sustained a concussion were three times more likely to suffer another *within the same season*.[21] Considering that as many as 60 percent of high school students may already have sustained at least one brain injury, it appears that a growing population of young athletes may experience as yet undiagnosed cognitive impairment later in life.[22] Perhaps the scariest bit, however, is that we just don't know how many concussions it might take to trigger conditions such as dementia; depression; or CTE, a devastating form of brain degeneration that's been discovered in the brains of more than fifty former professional athletes, as well as in the brain of an eighteen-year-old (see this book's introduction for more on CTE).

Even before we began to fully understand the cumulative effects of multiple brain injuries, high schools and universities typically made some sort of effort to keep athletes with multiple concussions off the field. For example, lots of schools have enforced the "three strikes and you're out" rule: any athlete who sustains three concussions (typically over the course of a high school career) is no longer allowed to participate in school-sponsored sports. But these kinds of arbitrary guidelines have little basis in research, and aren't even particularly helpful or useful. Is the athlete who sustained two recent concussions and experienced lingering symptoms after each, for example, any more fit to continue playing than the athlete who sustained three concussions over a period of three years, and was asymptomatic within a few days each time?

But the real problem with this kind of arbitrary three-strikes rule is that athletes are rarely aware of exactly how many concussions they may already have sustained. In my own clinical research, my colleagues and I have often listened to children describe having felt the *symptoms* of concussion—a tackle that left them "seeing stars" or that gave them a pounding headache—yet they have no idea that they had actually sustained a brain injury. What's more, the parents of concussed children often have no idea that their child sustained an injury, either. Time after time, we've watched parents become both embarrassed and alarmed when their child begins listing—for the first time—the symptoms he or she felt after a hard hit or rough tackle. Therefore, it's actually quite likely that many athletes, especially those who have played their particular sport for several years, have experienced unidentified concussions at some point in the past.

EARLY RETIREMENT: WHEN CONTACT OR COLLISION SPORTS ARE NO LONGER WORTH THE RISK

Sometimes, particularly when an athlete has sustained multiple concussions or struggled with lingering symptoms for a period of months, returning to contact sports might *never* be advisable. Yet, deciding whether to continue playing is a complex question with no straight answer. As I've mentioned, there is no magic number to determine how many concussions are too many. Here are two hypothetical cases in which you might be forced to decide whether your child should continue with his or her chosen sport:

Your twelve-year-old hockey player already had long-standing attention or learning difficulties in school, and then he sustained three concussions over the course of two years, each of which resulted in headaches that lingered for weeks. In this instance, what can be gained from allowing him to continue playing? My suggestion: transition the child to a safer, limited- or non-contact sport.

If, on other hand, your athlete is an eighteen-year-old basketball player who suffered three concussions over a period of eight years (with no resulting amnesia or loss of consciousness, and a period of at least two years between each injury); had full, quick recoveries; had very strong post-concussion cognitive test scores (above the 80th percentile); experienced no residual symptoms or problems; and is extremely talented in the sport, with a desire to play in college and perhaps even professionally, then determining whether to continue playing becomes a much more complex decision.

Every athlete is different, and must be treated individually. If your child has sustained multiple concussions, or has experienced lingering post-concussion symptoms, there are several factors to consider before deciding whether to continue in organized athletics.

- *The timing of the concussions.* Did the concussions occur in the same calendar year? Three concussions spaced over a period of seventeen years are not necessarily the same as three concussions occurring within a single season.

- *The number and severity of post-concussion symptoms, and the length of recovery time.* The athlete who experienced post-concussion syndrome is not the same as the athlete who had a concussion in which symptoms resolved in less than a day or so, with no recurrence of those symptoms.

- *The nature of the sport.* Is your child's chosen sport considered a collision sport or a contact sport? Is the risk for injury high or low? A football player, for example, might be at greater risk of sustaining another injury than, say, a softball player.

- *The age of the athlete.* Perhaps not surprisingly, studies indicate that the longer a child participates in organized athletics, the greater the risk of eventual concussion. So if your child is only ten years old, but has already suffered three concussions, he has a greater chance of sustaining yet another injury over the remainder of his athletic career (which might span another eight to twelve years), than does, say, a college athlete, who might have only a year or so left to participate in school-sponsored sports. The more concussions a child sustains over a lifetime, the more likely he is to suffer long-term problems and cumulative cognitive damage.

- *The athlete's comfort level with concussion risk.* Is your child confident in her abilities and ready to continue playing, or does she feel anxiety about the chance of sustaining a further injury? Generally speaking, less confident players may actually put themselves at greater risk of injury during a game.

· *The athlete's behavior in practice or game play.* Is your child a risk taker on the field? Would you consider your child a "safe" or a "dangerous" player?

· *The athlete's genetic predisposition, learning or developmental disorders, or other "modifying factors."*[23] Although a possible genetic predisposition to concussion (the presence of ApoE4, for example) is still being researched, we do know that children with developmental concerns, including ADHD and learning disorders, tend to be at greater risk for concussion, tend to experience more severe and long-lasting symptoms, and tend to perform poorly on post-concussion neurocognitive testing.

· *The athlete's desire to continue playing.* How important is playing this sport for your child? If he's not very passionate about high school football, for example, and has no interest in playing in college and no desire (or ability) to consider a professional career, then why not choose another sport that carries less inherent risk? On the other hand, an extremely talented player who is banking on earning a college football scholarship or has aspirations to play in the NFL might be willing to take on additional risk in order to continue with the sport he loves. (I caution parents, however, that ultimately *they* are responsible for the safety of their kid's brains; sometimes, no matter how much a child loves to play, it just isn't safe to continue.)

Ultimately, all sports carry some inherent risk—and all of the factors I've noted, not just one, should be considered collectively to determine the level of risk for your particular child. Some parents simply don't believe in subjecting their children to *any* risk, and will avoid or forbid participation in all organized sports. Others feel that life itself carries inherent risk, and don't believe in missing out on the benefits of sports *just in case* an injury might occur. But regardless of how you feel personally, I can tell you that the absolute hardest part of my job is conveying the news that a child athlete needs to stop playing his or her chosen sport.

It's easy to overlook the hold that sports have on our children. Organized athletics—with the accompanying social network, the friends, the travel, the games, and the joy of winning and working together as a team—have a tendency to define who we are as individuals, and even as families (because parents of athletic children often form close friendships, too). The stress of losing all that is what sometimes drives children to become so angry and emotional—even more than might be typical, due to the chemical changes in their concussed brains—that they cry, yell, scream, throw tantrums, and proclaim that they'll *never* give up their sport, no matter what the cost. And it pains me to watch parents struggle to make the best choice for their child. It's easier, certainly, to be in denial about the long-term risks of multiple concussions than to face reality, so stressed-out parents sometimes "shop" for doctors who will tell them what they want to hear. There are parents who try desperately to convince themselves—and their doctors—that another concussion "won't happen to them," or that their children will defy the odds. Yet these well-meaning, well-intentioned parents are gambling with their children's lives.

My hope is that, by reading this book, you may learn to monitor your child's brain hygiene (see Chapter 7) and sports activity so that you never find yourself in this kind of emotional predicament. The concussed athletes who fare best when faced with the decision to stop a particular sport are generally those who enjoy other low-risk sports, who have other interests and endeavors (not just athletic), who have strong self-esteem, clear academic goals, and an understanding that the brain is too precious to jeopardize. And they generally have assertive parents who are able to make the responsible choice and support the change. If your child has a passion for a specific contact sport, encourage him to also participate in and develop a skill set in a non-contact sport. He'll become a more well-rounded athlete, and will have something to fall back on if he develops a history of concussion.

Make sure that your child's school or youth sports league reinforces the message of brain hygiene and concussion education. I don't recommend scare tactics; a healthy, normalized approach—just as we take with dental hygiene or personal care—is best. And if your child does sustain a concussion, be sure to seek care from a licensed health care provider. You may best reduce the risk of future concussions and the probability of having to end participation in sports by managing each concussion carefully, without trying to rush the recovery period. Comply with your doctor's instructions. If you believe in the team of professionals involved with your child's care, then your child is more likely to as well. If you waver, it will be more difficult for your child to comply with rest and recovery.

Chapter 5 Review

- · When in doubt, sit them out. Compared to adults, youth athletes need more time to heal from concussions. Sending your child back to play too soon can put her at risk for a catastrophic, even deadly injury.

- · Although no helmet or mouth guard can completely eliminate the risk of concussion, you should ensure that your child is using the best equipment available, and that his equipment has been reconditioned properly and recently.

- · The effects of multiple concussions can compound over time. Children who have had two, three, or more concussions are more likely to experience long-term cognitive, emotional, and behavioral problems.

- · There is no magic number of concussions to determine when an athlete should no longer participate in his chosen sport.

Whether to continue playing is a complex question with no straight answer, and the inherent risks should be discussed within the family, with help and guidance from your circle of health care providers.

DRAFTING A CONCUSSION
HEALTH CARE TEAM

Lindsey was just thirteen years old when she sustained her first concussion. During a basketball game at her Pennsylvania middle school, she leaped over an opposing player who had fallen to the ground. In midair, that opponent reached out and grabbed Lindsey's ankle and—*whack!*—Lindsey's head went slamming against the floor. Despite the dizziness, balance problems, screaming headache, and nausea, she might have been fine had she been given appropriate time to rest and recover. Unfortunately, Lindsey suffered her second concussion just two weeks later (basketball again—an errant elbow to the head). One week after *that*, she'd already earned her third.

Over the course of the following year, Lindsey sank deeper and deeper into the grip of post-concussion syndrome, or PCS. Not that her parents, her teachers, or her coach had any idea; Lindsey had never had a baseline test, her school had no concussion identification or management policy, and her parents—in the absence of any real education—mistakenly thought that Lindsey's "injuries" weren't much more than bumps on the head. And yet, Lindsey was clearly not the same. She was irrational, irritable, and argumentative. Her out-of-control emotions had driven away her friends, and within a few months' time, she'd become isolated and alone. By the time Lindsey's impulsive behavior had earned her not one, but two suspensions from school, her mother was pretty much beside herself. Lindsey, after all, had been a straight-A student with zero history of disciplinary problems. Now—her mother thought—she was barely recognizable. It wasn't until Lindsey's *fourth* concussion (sustained about a year after her third) that someone finally referred her to a neuropsychologist. That doctor, it turns out, was me.

Concussions, as I hope I've now made quite clear, are elusive injuries, and they're difficult to diagnose. Remember, there is no single specific test—no CT scan or X-ray, no blood screening or exercise—that can definitively pinpoint a mild brain injury, or can help a doctor determine, within a day or two of impact, exactly how long it will take before the patient fully recovers. In Lindsey's case, her family doctor *did* order an MRI shortly after her third concussion. When the results came back normal, however, that was the end of that. Without a second opinion or a concussion-management program to follow, Lindsey was left to languish for months and months and months. In other words, Lindsey's case had fallen through the cracks.

I wish I could say that what happened to Lindsey is a rare and random occurrence. Unfortunately, this kind of thing happens all too often. The elusiveness of concussion—the ambiguity of the injury—is precisely why so many of them go unnoticed and untreated. And when health care providers aren't encouraged to work *together*, parents often find themselves drifting from one doctor to the next without ever really getting the help they need. After Lindsey's third concussion, for example, a doctor in the local emergency room suggested she see a neuropsychologist, but didn't know of any in the area that treated children. A psychiatrist would later recommend a consultation with a brain trauma specialist, but her parents thought that seemed a bit extreme. Ultimately, Lindsey was put on the antianxiety medication Zoloft (to help with her emotional distress), but it would be another six months before she found her way to me.

Lindsey's story may be an exercise in what-ifs: What if her school had a consulting neuropsychologist in place? What if her parents had taken the psychiatrist's advice? But it's also an example of the need to draft a concussion health care *team,* and to have that team in place before an in-jury occurs. By consulting with a group of medical specialists with varying backgrounds—specialists who have been trained to manage brain inju-ries and have experience working as a unit—you increase the likelihood of catching an undiagnosed concussion, and you lessen the likelihood of returning an injured athlete to play too soon. And when one of those ex-perts isn't so easy to track down—perhaps your insurance won't cover a neuropsychological visit, or your child's school doesn't employ an athletic trainer—the other members of the team can step up to the plate.

Generally speaking, a good concussion health care team should consist of three key members: (1) a family or school doctor or pediatrician (who can perform an initial medical exam and, if needed, order CT scans or MRIS to rule out other, more serious injuries); (2) a neuropsychologist (to ad-minister post-concussion testing and monitor the athlete's cognitive re-covery); and (3) an athletic trainer (to perform physical exertional testing and guide the athlete through a step-by-step return to physical activity). But there are other adults who will play an integral role in your child's athletic career, and it's important that *all* of them have been trained to recognize the signs and symptoms of a brain injury. Here's what you need to know about getting your concussion health care team in place.

THE COACH

Perhaps more than any other adult in your child's athletic life, it's the coach who will set the tone for both success and safety in sports. A good coach promotes fair play, employs constructive criticism, and never re-sorts to bullying or intimidation. A good coach focuses on building con-fidence and camaraderie among the players, and always puts the health and safety of athletes first. Luckily, there are hundreds of thousands of excellent youth and amateur coaches across the country, men and women whose primary focus is not *just* on winning, but on cultivating a love of the game, too. Unfortunately, many of these coaches haven't received any kind of concussion management or treatment training, nor have they been taught the signs and symptoms of brain injury. In a 2010 survey of parents whose children (ages twelve to seventeen) participate in school-sponsored sports, researchers at C. S. Mott Children's Hospital and the University of Michigan discovered that 50 percent of respondents knew a coach who would return athletes to play too soon.[1]

Some states have attempted to address these concerns by passing legislation that requires youth athletic coaches to undergo specific concussion-management training each and every year. The vast majority of the new concussion laws, however, do *not* mandate training for coaches; and even those that do often pertain only to school-sponsored athletics. This means that if your child plays for a community or youth league, there's an even greater likelihood that his or her coach has not received training about identifying concussions in kids.

Questions to Ask Your Child's Coach

· Does the team have a formal concussion-management program in place? Are parents required to provide formal, written, informed consent regarding concussion risk before youth athletes are allowed to play?

· Do you educate your players about the dangers of concussion? Do you encourage them to report the signs and symptoms (both their own and their teammates')?

· What kind of health care professionals are available to my child during practices and games? Does the team travel with a certified athletic trainer?

· If my child sustains a concussion, will he be required to leave the game? What steps, if any, must he take before he is cleared to return to play?

· What happens if my child sustains a concussion at an *away* game? Will he be sent to a local hospital? Examined by an athletic trainer or physician?

Did You Know . . . ?

Coaches who violate statewide concussion laws in Connecticut may have their coaching permits revoked by the board of education. Connecticut Senate Bill 456, signed into law in May 2010, mandates that any concussed athlete must be immediately removed from play, and requires coaches to take yearly refresher courses on concussion identification and management. Unfortunately, the vast majority of state laws do *not* require training or certification for youth and amateur coaches. To access a free online concussion course for coaches (Heads Up), log on to the US Centers for Disease Control and Prevention website (www.cdc.gov/concussion/).

· What kind of helmets and protective athletic equipment do the players use? How often is that equipment reconditioned or recertified?

THE CERTIFIED ATHLETIC TRAINER

A certified athletic trainer (ATC) is a health care specialist with training in injury prevention, recognition, and rehabilitation. He or she is often the first line of defense in the management of concussions. After all, it's usually an athletic trainer (rather than, say, a physician) who is present on the sidelines during practices and games. It's often the responsibility of the athletic trainer, rather than a coach, to determine when and if an injured athlete should be removed from play. And when a potentially more catastrophic injury occurs, it's usually the athletic trainer who is best suited to summon an ambulance and communicate with paramedics, nurses, and doctors.

In the event that your child sustains a concussion, the athletic trainer becomes fundamental in the recovery process and return-to-play decision. Athletic trainers are the best suited to administer sideline assessment tests—such as the Sport Concussion Assessment Tool (SCAT2; see Chapter 4) or Standardized Assessment of Concussion (SAC; see Chap-

Did You Know . . . ?

In some states, organizations from the private sector are step-ping up to fill the concussion health care void. The Carolinas Medical Center hospital system in Charlotte, North Carolina, for example, began providing free athletic trainers to local high schools, partly in the hope of drumming up business.[3] If your child plays for a team without an athletic trainer, don't hesi-tate to contact private sports medicine clinics or hospitals in your area.

ter 2)—to document the immediate signs and symptoms. And during the recovery process, it's the athletic trainer who should conduct physi-cal exertional testing, as well as guide the athlete through a step-by-step return to play.

Unfortunately, fewer than half of American high schools have access to an athletic trainer, and the chance is even lower that your child's ele-mentary or middle school, or community or recreation league, has access to one.[2] Some schools are able to provide an athletic trainer for games only; some, in the absence of a trainer, will hire a consulting physician. If your child is playing for a school, club sport, or recreation league without an athletic trainer in place, you may want to speak to your child's coach, athletic director, or principal about adding an athletic trainer to the staff as soon as possible. If that doesn't work, consider contacting the board of education or attending a school board meeting in your district. There is a movement afoot to *require* schools, particularly high schools, to hire cer-tified athletic trainers, but that's unlikely to happen unless parents be-come more vocal and start insisting on better care for their children.

Youth and recreation leagues rarely have the funding in place to hire athletic trainers, so partnering with other parents and organizing a fund-raiser may prove helpful. Then, contact a sports medicine clinic or local hospital and ask about hiring an athletic trainer or volunteer interns on a part-time basis. Be sure that anyone you contact has expertise and train-ing in concussions, specifically.

Questions to Ask Your Child's Certified Athletic Trainer

· Is there a baseline neurocognitive testing program in place? If so, what version of the test is used (for example, the newer, online version of IMPACT; older, desktop version of IMPACT; Axon Sports Computerized Cognitive Assessment Tool; HeadMinder Concussion Resolution Index)?

· How is the baseline testing performed? Are youth athletes tested in groups or individually? Are the baseline scores reviewed by a neurocognitive specialist? How often are the baseline tests updated, if ever?

· Does the athletic program consult with a neuropsychologist or other neurocognitive specialist for help with return-to-play decisions?

· If my child sustains a concussion, what steps must she take before being allowed to return to play?

· Does the athletic training department use physical exertional testing and a step-by-step return-to-play protocol for concussed athletes?

THE SCHOOL NURSE

We already know that very young children are more likely to sustain concussions during free play or recess than while competing in organized athletics. If your child isn't yet of high school age, know that you'll likely find a nurse—rather than an athletic trainer—in charge of concussion programs and return-to-play clearances at school (rarely do elementary and middle schools add an athletic trainer to their full-time staff). School nurses, however, tend to function similarly to athletic trainers when it comes to concussion management; they may be called upon to administer preseason baseline testing, and to monitor an injured child's return to both the classroom and sports. Make sure that your child's school nurse is up to date on concussion guidelines and understands that brain injuries are not just caused by blows to the head—a fall on the playground, for example, could leave a youngster in much the same condition as would a rough tackle on the football field.

Questions to Ask Your Child's School Nurse

· Does the school have a concussion-management policy in place? Will my child be sent to the nurse's office as soon as someone *suspects* he might have sustained a concussion?

· Do you keep a concussion signs and symptoms checklist in your office? The Acute Concussion Evaluation (ACE) form is sometimes used by schools not only to document concussion, but to check off the recommendations for academic accommodations, physical exertional testing, and return to play. If your school nurse doesn't have access to the ACE form, you can find one on the CDC website (see Appendix A for the web address).

· Do you keep a record of any injuries that might occur during free play or recess, and will you notify me if my child gets hurt, even if the injury doesn't appear serious?

· Have you worked with any concussed students who were granted academic accommodations during their recovery? Does the school have a working relationship with a neuro-psychologist or concussion specialist?

THE EMERGENCY ROOM PHYSICIAN, FAMILY OR SCHOOL DOCTOR, AND PEDIATRICIAN

Although a large number of ER physicians, family and school doctors, and pediatricians may not be up to date on the latest concussion-management guidelines, these kinds of doctors still play an integral role in the identification and recovery process. That's because any child who has sustained a possible concussion should be examined by a physician to rule out a more serious injury. Depending on the type and severity of your child's symptoms, the doctor may order a CT scan or MRI. (But remember, any doctor who tells you that your child didn't sustain a concussion because the CT scan was "normal" is misinformed.) Additionally, some new statewide concussion laws mandate that a physician—rather than a neuropsychologist—is required to provide the final written return-to-play clearance after the concussed athlete has recovered. If that's the case in your state, make sure that your child's physician has consulted with a neuropsychologist before allowing your child back on the field.

Questions to Ask Your Child's Physician

· Do you have training and experience in treating concussions based on the most recent management and return-to-play guidelines?

· Does my child need a CT scan or MRI to rule out something more than a concussion?

· Should I wake up my child periodically throughout the night after she sustains a concussion? (Though most concussed children do *not* need to be awakened periodically—sleep is necessary for the brain to heal itself—each brain injury is different, so it's always best to ask.)

· Will you be available to communicate with my child's neuropsychologist and other health care team specialists regarding her post-concussion testing results and recovery process?

· What steps should my child take, or what will you require my child to do (or not do), before you can provide written return-to-play clearance?

THE NEUROPSYCHOLOGIST

Neuropsychologists, or brain-behavior specialists, are doctoral-level health care professionals who have typically completed a four-year undergraduate degree, a four- to six-year graduate degree in psychology with a specialization in neuropsychology, and at least two years of supervised clinical training followed by national exam and state exam and licensure. They are trained to understand what happens when the brain is injured, and are the best suited to interpret preseason and post-concussion tests. And although it's not mandatory, many neuropsychologists are board certified—through additional examination—to further demonstrate their professional expertise. But let's be honest: it's pretty unlikely that your child's school has a neuropsychologist on staff. Instead, most schools rely on an athletic trainer alone to administer baseline testing, without neuropsychological consultation. Athletic trainers are also often called upon to interpret post-concussion testing, even though they are not trained or qualified neurocognitive specialists. And of course, that's assuming your child's school even offers neurocognitive testing in the first place.

Ideally, all schools and community sports organizations should have some kind of affiliation with a neuropsychologist in the area. That way, athletic trainers have someone available to verify and validate baseline test scores, as well as someone to collaborate and consult with during an athlete's individual return-to-play process. Ask your child's coach, athletic trainer, or athletic director if the school has a consulting neuro-psychologist or concussion-management team in place. (With the passage of new statewide concussion laws, more and more schools are, in fact, securing consulting relationships with neuropsychologists.) And if it doesn't, urge the school to forge a partnership. (I consult with several youth leagues and schools in my area, including a few sprawling hockey associations that have made commitments to baseline all athletes above the age of ten as part of yearly registration.) If your school or community sports league won't budge, consider securing private baseline testing from a neuropsychologist in your area—that way you'll be ready before an injury even occurs.

Questions to Ask Your Child's Neuropsychologist

· Do you have experience interpreting baseline and post-concussion neurocognitive testing? If so, what version or brand of testing do you use in your office?

· How soon after an injury should a child undergo post-concussion neurocognitive testing? How often do you recommend repeating the test before determining if a child has fully recovered?

· Will you be available to communicate with my child's doctor or athletic trainer regarding physical exertional testing and a step-by-step return-to-play protocol?

· Do you have experience creating custom academic plans for youth athletes with lingering concussion symptoms? Do you have experience communicating with school personnel about the necessity of implementing academic accommodations?

· What steps should my child take, or what will you require my child to do (or not do), before you can provide written return-to-play clearance?

· Can you refer my child to a neurologist, biofeedback specialist, or other medical specialist in the event that he develops PCS? Do you have experience recommending or administering alternative therapies?

TACKLING COMMUNITY SPORTS LEAGUES

While schools across the country are scrambling to get official concussion-management programs in place, community-based and recreation sports leagues are largely being left in the lurch—that's because the

Case Study No. 3

PATIENT: Lindsey, fifteen-year-old female

PREFERRED SPORT: Basketball (school and private youth league)

FIRST APPOINTMENT WITH DR. MOSER: February 2011 (age fourteen)

TYPE OF AND DATE(S) OF INJURY:

Concussion 1: Age thirteen. During a middle school basketball game, Lindsey jumped over an opposing player who had fallen to the ground. The player grabbed Lindsey's ankle; she fell, and slammed her head into the floor. *Immediate symptoms*: Dizziness, confusion, possible amnesia, balance problems, headache, nausea. Lindsey was kept out of gym class for four days and avoided basketball for two weeks. No other restrictions. No outside medical supervision.

Concussion 2: Age thirteen; two weeks later. During a youth league basketball game, Lindsey was attempting to rebound the ball when an opposing player's elbow collided with her head. *Immediate symptoms*: Headache, possible amnesia. Lindsey was removed from play and kept out of sports for two weeks. No other restrictions.

Concussion 3: Age thirteen; one week later. During an exercise in gym class, Lindsey became dizzy, fell to the floor, and hit her head. *Immediate symptoms*: Brief loss of consciousness, headache. Lindsey was taken to the local ER, but the doctor did not perform a CT scan. Her family doctor ordered an MRI, but the results were normal. Ultimately, she was put on antianxiety medication for "unexplained" behavioral and disciplinary issues.

Concussion 4: Age fourteen; approximately one year later. Lindsey tripped and fell during a youth league basketball game, hitting her head on the floor. *Immediate symptoms*: Headache. Lindsey's first appointment with me was the next day.

INITIAL EXAM: By the time Lindsey came to see me (she was referred by another patient, a fellow student at her school), her symptoms were many: memory loss, anxiety, irritability,

(continued)

(continued)

impulsivity, mental slowness, and fatigue. Her family was completely confused by the change in her behavior; her mother described the symptoms as having come on "like a storm." Even Lindsey herself couldn't explain why her life had changed so much in the previous thirteen months. When her mother had asked other doctors if concussions could be to blame, none could offer her an answer.

Because Lindsey had never had a neurocognitive baseline established, I had her sit for ImPACT testing at her first appointment. Her total symptom score (which, for most children, ranges from 0 to 4), was 36. On tests of verbal memory and visual memory, she scored *below the first percentile*. I also referred her to a neurologist for additional consultation (exams came back unremarkable).

RECOVERY PLAN: Complete mental and physical rest for two full weeks: no school, no computers, no texting, no reading, no homework, no chores, no exercise, no leaving the house for shopping, no socializing, no guests. Mild television and minimal cell phone use. Extra sleep. Medical report and recommendations were sent to Lindsey's school. Both she and her mother were very skeptical of these recommendations. After the initial two-week recovery period, however, Lindsey showed dramatic improvement in ImPACT scores. She was returned to school on a half-day basis the following week.

At the end of the third week, Lindsey's condition had improved enough to try physical exertional testing (she passed). She was then reconditioned to exercise under the supervision of a certified athletic trainer. By the eighth week, Lindsey felt "awesome," and she was cleared to return to sports by consensus of her physician, her athletic trainer, and myself; her health care team recommended low-contact/low-risk activities.

ACADEMIC ACCOMMODATIONS: Luckily, Lindsey's school was incredibly accommodating during her recovery process. She was excused from all homework and in-class testing, as well as from statewide standardized testing (the Pennsylvania System of School Assessment test, or PSSA) and gym class. She was *not* required to make up any lost work. After three weeks of half-days, she returned to school full time.

NOTES: Except for a study my colleagues and I completed,[4] there is little research to confirm the effectiveness of rest when applied months after injury (ideally, an injured athlete would start a course of rest immediately). But in Lindsey's case, a few weeks of rest made all the difference in the world—her ImPACT scores improved *dramatically*, with some scores reaching the 97th to 99th percentile.

ImPACT Results

	Initial Exam	Second Exam (2 weeks later)	Final Exam (8 weeks later)
Verbal memory	<1%	85%	97%
Visual memory	1%	63%	99%
Visual-motor speed	17%	34%	35%
Reaction time	16%	38%	64%
Total symptoms	36	4	1

NOTES FROM LINDSEY'S MOM: "The year that my daughter had post-concussion syndrome was one of the most difficult years of my life. I knew the emotional pulse of my child had changed dramatically and almost overnight, but none of the doctors we saw could help us. It's horrible to watch your child suffer and not understand why, to not be able to help them.

"When Lindsey and I first saw Dr. Moser, we were skeptical that *rest* could really be the solution to our yearlong saga. But I was amazed at just how much she slept once her brain was allowed to shut off—she averaged twelve hours a night, with two- to three-hour naps throughout the day. The change in her demeanor was incredible; it was like I got my daughter back.

"If there's any advice I have for parents of child athletes, it's this: Educate yourself about the dangers of concussion. Make sure that your school or community sports organization has a concussion-management policy in place. If she does get hurt, see a professional immediately (one that deals specifically with identification and management of brain injuries). And never think that a concussion is just a bump on the head. One of my greatest regrets is that we didn't find a neuropsychologist sooner—we might have saved our whole family a lot of stress and sadness if we had."

vast majority of new concussion laws do not extend beyond interscholastic athletics, and many do not cover student athletes until they reach high school age. If you've got a youngster playing in a private athletic league, then he may still be vulnerable to suffering an unrecognized or misdiagnosed concussion; he may be less likely to get the treatment he needs. So make sure that your child's prospective coach has a plan in place *before* you sign up your kid for fall football or spring soccer. Here's what you need to know about the challenges facing non-school-based athletic leagues:

- Community-based and recreation sports leagues are often run by parents and volunteer coaches, the vast majority of whom have little or no formal experience or training. In fact, 85 percent of youth athletic coaches are fathers coaching their own children.[5] That means it's often left to parents to create a concussion-management program; to make sure coaches and officials have been trained to identify the signs and symptoms of a brain injury; and to forge relationships with doctors, neuropsychologists, athletic trainers, and other concussion experts in the area.

- Small, neighborhood-oriented organizations may have greater difficulties funding concussion-management programs. While some of the nation's largest private athletic leagues, including Pop Warner football and USA Hockey, are already changing the way they respond to brain injuries (by requiring injured athletes to sit the bench, for example, and insisting on written medical clearance before a return to play), smaller local leagues may not have the knowledge base to mandate those kinds of rules. The chances are even lower that a local team will have the funding to provide preseason baseline testing, or to set up a working relationship with a neuropsychologist in the area. But just as parents can band together to secure better-quality helmets and athletic equipment for their children, they can join forces to organize group-rate or discounted neurocognitive testing, or to invite a concussion specialist to educate parents about brain injuries—or do both! And in fact, most youth leagues will welcome with open arms this kind of parental involvement.

· Community or club athletic coaches rarely have any communication with an athlete's teachers, school nurse, or athletic trainer. If your child sustained a concussion during a high school football game, his coach will probably communicate this to an athletic trainer, a school nurse, a guidance counselor, or some other staff member. (After all, these individuals are employed at the same place.) If your child is injured during a non-school-league game, however, it's unlikely that his teachers or athletic trainers would have any knowledge of the event. No matter what, your child's teachers and guidance counselor still need to know about any concussions—regardless of when or where they occurred—to be able to monitor your child's recovery, watch out for worsening symptoms, and help facilitate any academic accommodations. Keep the communication lines open at all times.

Chapter 6 Review

· Don't wait to draft a concussion health care team—make sure all the adults in your child's athletic life are up to date on concussion identification and management, and are prepared to work together to spot an injury *before* one ever occurs.

· Even if your school doesn't have an athletic trainer or neurocognitive specialist on staff, it's possible to partner with sports medicine clinics, local hospitals, or other private medical experts to secure any concussion oversight your team may need. Don't be afraid to draft your own team of experts, rather than expecting a school or youth sports organization to do it for you. You can contact your state brain injury association for support, resources, and available grants.

· If your child sustains a concussion during a non-school-based practice or game, don't hesitate to share that information with teachers, athletic trainers, and nurses at your child's school.

CHANGING THE GAME

Public Education, Advocacy, and the Brain Hygiene Model

In late July 2011, seventy-five former professional football players, along with some former players' wives, filed suit against the National Football League. Among the allegations in the eighty-six-page document filed with Los Angeles County Superior Court? That the NFL knew about the long-term effects of multiple concussions, yet "willfully, wantonly, egregiously . . . and with a high degree of moral culpability" deceived its players, coaches, and trainers for more than eighty years; that the NFL knew its players were at risk for brain damage, dementia, depression, and even death, and yet did nothing to stop it.[1]

Perhaps not surprisingly, spokespersons for the NFL, in the days following the announcement of the class-action lawsuit, promised that the league would "vigorously contest any claims" of wrongdoing.[1] But what *is* surprising, as well as particularly telling of the current state of concussion awareness in this country, has been the response from the general public. On hundreds of message boards and forums across the Internet, fans have decried the lawsuit as baseless, frivolous, silly, and even shameful. Some have labeled it a simple money grab, while others have likened it to the infamous "hot coffee" lawsuit of 1994, otherwise known as *Liebeck vs. McDonald's Restaurants*, the case of a seventy-nine-year-old woman who successfully sued McDonald's after burning herself with a scalding cup of coffee, inciting a heated tort reform debate in the process.[2]

But it's this comment, posted on the *Palm Beach Post* website on July 21, 2011, that perhaps best sums up the contrarian view:

> So your [*sic*] gonna tell me these 75 former players are suing because they weren't told how dangerous it is to beat the tar outta one another? Thank God for football because these 75 players are too stupid to have done anything else.[3]

The subtext of such messages is clear: football carries an inherent risk of injury; shouldn't athletes *expect* to get injured at some point? But the heart of the issue isn't so much whether the NFL properly informed its players of the dangers of concussion, it's whether the NFL knew about these dangers and then *denied them*. After all, doctors from the NFL's own Mild Traumatic Brain Injury Committee, established in 1994 to study the long-term effects of concussion, vehemently contested Dr. Bennet Omalu's discovery of chronic traumatic encephalopathy in the brain of "Iron Mike" Webster. They called Omalu's findings "seriously flawed" and petitioned the editor of *Neurosurgery* to retract Omalu's published article. (He did not.)[4] The following year, two of these doctors—David Viano and Elliot Pellman—published their own research in the journal *Neurosurgical Focus*. In what amounted to a rebuttal of Omalu's findings, Viano and Pellman claimed that "mild [traumatic brain injuries] in professional football are not serious injuries," largely based on the fact that most concussed players returned to the game within a week.[5, 6] (Most concussion experts would surely find this position illogical as well as irresponsible.)

By 2007, amid a growing flurry of negative publicity, the NFL had begun taking *some* steps to address brain injuries. Commissioner Roger Goodell ordered mandatory baseline neurocognitive testing for every NFL athlete, and also announced the creation of the 88 Plan, named in honor of Hall of Famer John Mackey—number 88 for the Baltimore Colts—who was diagnosed with dementia in 2001 at the age of 59. The 88 Plan provides up to $88,000 per year for ex-players suffering from dementia or Alzheimer's, but NFL officials were quick to point out that

> ### Did You Know . . . ?
>
> Dr. Gay Culverhouse, former president of the Tampa Bay Buc-
> caneers and author of *Throwaway Players: The Concussion
> Crisis*, founded the Gay Culverhouse Player's Outreach Pro-
> gram to help retired NFL players access health care and dis-
> ability benefits. "I work with players who are homeless now
> and so demented we can't get them to understand the ser-
> vices that are available to them," she told Tampa Bay Online.[13]
> To date, the program has identified two dozen former players
> who may be entitled to union benefits, as well as being paid
> for their necessary medical exams.[14] Read more about her
> progress at www.playersoutreach.org.

such diseases aren't necessarily indicative of concussions, and may well be the result of old age. "It's a matter of addressing a need, without re-gard to cause or circumstances," NFL spokesman Greg Aiello told the Associated Press.[7]

Despite these small steps, however, the NFL still wasn't buying the link between concussions and long-term damage—at least not publicly. Following its first annual Concussion Summit in June 2007, Ira Casson, co-chairman of the NFL's Mild Traumatic Brain Injury Committee, told reporters that "the only scientifically valid evidence of chronic encephal-opathy in athletes is in boxers and in some steeplechase jockeys. It's never been scientifically, validly documented in any other athletes."[8] (Never mind the fact that Omalu had already discovered evidence of CTE in at least three other deceased players' brains, to say nothing of the other research studies that indicated a link between multiple concussions and clinical depression, as well as an increased risk of Alzheimer's disease.) And in a pamphlet dated August 14, 2007, players were told that "cur-rent research with professional athletes has not shown that having more than one or two concussions leads to permanent problems if each injury is treated properly."[9, 10]

It wasn't until late 2009 that the NFL began to radically change its tune. New league-wide policy barred the same-day return to play of concussed athletes, and posters went up in every NFL locker room across the country, declaring that "traumatic brain injury . . . may lead to problems with memory and communication, personality changes, as well as depression and the early onset of dementia.[11] Concussions and conditions resulting from repeated brain injury can change your life and your family's life forever."[12] It's this sudden reversal of position that is the crux of the former players' 2011 class-action lawsuit.

Regardless of how you feel about the lawsuit, its existence is further proof that we are in the midst of both a heated concussion debate and a sweeping cultural shift. And it's the NFL, interestingly enough, that has begun to lead the charge. Aside from levying huge fines against players committing "dangerous," concussion-inducing tackles, the NFL has retooled its Mild Traumatic Brain Injury Committee—and doctors Casson, Viano, and Pellman will not be serving as members of the newly named Head, Neck, and Spine Committee.[13] Commissioner Goodell himself lobbied Congress and urged governors of all fifty states to pass youth concussion prevention legislation. To that end, he's been largely successful—thirty-four states have passed some form of youth concussion legislation since the state of Washington enacted the first-of-its-kind Zackery Lystedt Law in May 2009. (Many other states have legislation pending.)

Recall that Zackery Lystedt (see Chapter 1) was just thirteen when he developed second impact syndrome after returning to play too soon following a football-induced concussion. Washington State's House Bill 1824 and Senate Bill 5763—the legislation named for Lystedt—are considered model legislation for similar laws, and contain three important tenets (laws that do not contain all three tenets are considered weak by concussion experts and legislative advocates):

1. *Education.* Athletes, parents, and coaches must be educated on the signs, symptoms, and dangers of concussion.
2. *Removal from play.* Players who are suspected of having sustained a concussion must be immediately removed from play.

> ### Did You Know . . . ?
>
> Pro Football Hall of Famer Harry Carson, a former linebacker for the New York Giants, estimates that he suffered at least fifteen concussions over the course of his professional career. "One problem [with post-concussion syndrome] is that a lot of players who suffer from it have no clue what they're dealing with," he told *Sports Illustrated* in 2001.[16] "I've talked to players I've played with and against. Once I went public with this concussion thing, they were looking at me as being sort of brain-damaged, drooling and all this stuff. But it is an injury just like one to your knee or hip." Carson wrote at length about his struggles with PCS in his autobiography *Captain for Life: My Story as a Hall of Fame Linebacker*, published in 2011.

3. *Written medical clearance.* Concussed athletes are not permitted to return to play without written medical clearance from a licensed health care professional.

A duo of federal bills has been proposed as well. Rep. Bill Pascrell of New Jersey introduced HR 1347, the Concussion Treatment and Care Tools Act (CONTACT), which was passed by the House of Representatives in September 2010 but failed to clear the Senate (perhaps due largely to the economic downturn). HR 469, the Protecting Student Athletes from Concussions Act of 2011, was introduced in January 2011 and, at the time of this writing, has been referred to a committee for further review and debate.

In lieu of the passage of proposed federal legislation, several members of Congress, including Rep. Bill Pascrell, have charged the US Centers for Disease Control and Prevention with developing national guidelines for managing sports-related concussion. In September 2011, the CDC announced that it would convene a panel of experts to review current scientific literature. National protocols should be available for distribution by late 2014.

I am a devoted concussion legislation advocate—I was part of a team that presented the findings of the 2008 International Conference on Psychological Health and Traumatic Brain Injury to Congress, and I have lobbied for increased funding in the area of traumatic brain injury alongside Rep. Pascrell. Yet I also know that concussion legislation is not a cure-all. Legislation isn't much use without education on the signs, symptoms, and dangers of concussion, as well as a change in the current culture of collision and contact sports. (You can find a detailed, state-by-state overview of the most recent concussion legislation in Appendix E of this book.)

CULTURE WARS

These recent legislative efforts, combined with a series of multimillion-dollar lawsuits brought by the victims of concussion-related injuries, have sent ripples through professional sports, but also—and significantly—through youth and amateur leagues. The Pop Warner youth football league, for example, recently adopted more stringent concussion-management guidelines and announced the formation of its first medical advisory board. Months later, the Ivy League made some changes, too, announcing that it would limit the number of weekly full-contact football practices, decreasing it from the National Collegiate Athletic Association's maximum of five down to just two, in an attempt to reduce the number of hits that players sustain over the course of a season.[17]

Of course, changes like these are not just confined to amateur and professional football. The National Hockey League recently announced the creation of Rule 48, which slaps any athlete who targets the head of another player—when approaching from the lateral, or blind side—with a penalty. (By the start of the 2011–2012 season, that rule was further tweaked, eliminating targeted hits to the head from *any* direction.) And in response to the youth concussion crisis, USA Hockey raised the age at which in-game checking is allowed from the peewee level (ages eleven to twelve) to bantam level (ages thirteen to fourteen). That move was largely based on a growing body of research about the rate at which young players get injured on the ice. For example, Dr. Carolyn Emery of the University of Calgary in Alberta, Canada, studied youth hockey players for four years, and found that eleven- and twelve-year-olds who are allowed to check, when compared with those who are not, sustain four times as many concussions. At a 2010 Ice Hockey Summit, she explained that her research was "irrefutable evidence that delaying body checking until age 13 has significant benefits to the health of young players."[18]

In the face of that kind of research, barring body checks for young players might seem like a no-brainer. The decision, however, was not without controversy. Some, notably Dr. Barry Willer, a professor of psychiatry and rehabilitation medicine at the State University of New York–Buffalo, who has conducted his own research on the subject, have expressed concern that raising the age limit on in-game checking would actually *increase* the risk of injury to young players. The rule change, Willer told the *New York Times*, meant that thirteen-year-olds would have little or no experience giving a check, at an age when "there are big size discrepancies and a high level of testosterone."[19]

Others have opposed the rule change for a far simpler reason: eliminating checking renders the sport less recognizable, less like the game that fans are used to watching on television. If you're going to eliminate checking from hockey, fans have argued (with thinly veiled sarcasm), why not just eliminate tackling from football? In other words, how far are we going to go? In the wake of the rule change, some coaches even discussed flouting the rule altogether. "If we're allowed to go up [to Canada] and play hit hockey up there, we certainly will," Dan Dolan, a peewee coach in northern New York, told the *Buffalo News*.[20]

Indeed, it's this type of argument that points to the growing cultural rift among fans of contact and collision sports—the debate between keeping kids (and adults) safe, and maintaining the integrity of the game. The NFL met with its own fair share of drama when it began fining athletes for dangerous tackles; fans and players alike took this as a sign that the NFL had gone soft. "If you want to completely avoid health risks, maybe you shouldn't be playing this game," Seattle Seahawks linebacker Lofa

Did You Know . . . ?

Dr. Robert Cantu, co-director of the Center for the Study of Traumatic Encephalopathy at Boston University School of Medicine, recently recommended that children under age fourteen should not participate in collision sports as currently played, in light of recent research about the sensitivity of young brains and their vulnerability to concussion. But it is my opinion that we have a responsibility to make organized athletics as safe as possible for all children, regardless of their age. Preventing children from playing specific sports doesn't make those sports any safer when, as teenagers, kids do decide to participate. In fact, by the time a child reaches adolescence, his larger, stronger body may be more likely to inflict a concussive blow, especially if he's never been taught or practiced safe contact techniques.

I believe that by developing strong, school-based concussion awareness programs that begin educating young athletes at *very* early ages (kindergarten and up); by ensuring that youth coaches are educated in the most advanced, up-to-date safe training techniques; by promoting an atmosphere of zero tolerance for aggression and risky contact; by focusing more on skill development, especially when children's bodies are still small and lightweight (and therefore less able to inflict injury on fellow athletes); and by promoting reasonable game rule changes when appropriate, we may be more able to keep our kids safe, while also supporting long and successful athletic careers.

Tatupu told *GQ* magazine. "My dad [former Patriots running back Mosi Tatupu] played, and I look at the lifestyle it afforded me growing up . . . I know there's a risk, but to me all of this outweighs it."[21]

What is very, very easy to forget, though, is that the culture of most collision sports *has* changed considerably over time. In other words, what we see on television today, well, it ain't your father's football. For one thing, today's professional football players (as well as most other pro athletes) are giants compared to the men who used to play the game. Present-day offensive linemen, for example, weigh an average of 315 pounds,

65 pounds more than they did forty years ago.[22] Today's football stars wear less body padding, but are armed with helmets so dense that many have likened them to weapons. (Old-time players, with their soft shell of a helmet, were less likely to lead with their heads when tackling. Today's youth, on the other hand, are being taught to drill their opponents "right in his numbers," flying head-first at full speed.) That's to say nothing of the extreme pressures, both emotional and financial, that professional athletes face to keep playing, regardless of whether they're injured. (No pro athletes in the 1960s, 1970s, or early 1980s were making anything close to the multimillion-dollar contracts we read about today, not even when adjusted for inflation. *That* kind of money, and the threat of losing it by being sidelined with an injury, is serious motivation to suck it up and play though the pain.)

To assume that kind of cultural shift doesn't trickle down to amateur and youth leagues would be a mistake. Youth athletes idolize—and emulate—the players they see on television. They watch one pro athlete after another brush himself off after a bone-crunching tackle (often oblivious to the real repercussions of such forceful collisions), and they take that same kind of invincible, no-fear, hot-shot attitude back to high school and middle school football fields across the country. Christian Koelling, president of the Minnesota-based Duluth Amateur Hockey Association, has noticed these same kinds of style-of-play changes in youth hockey players: "Now you see more hits and more hits with injury potential," he told the *Star Tribune*. "Body contact at a young level should be 100 percent intended to gain possession of the puck. But there has been a shift in culture . . . [Checking] is used as intimidation."[23]

Contrary to what some die-hard fans may fear, however, most concussion experts don't advocate for taking the tackling out of football, or for turning hockey into a sport resembling figure skating. (In fact, many of the concussion experts and legislative advocates I work with are die-hard sports fans themselves.) The goal, rather, is to *prolong* each player's athletic career, and to lessen the chance of both acute and long-term injury. To do that effectively, we have to take an objective look at all possible options—things like stricter return-to-play guidelines, safer and more advanced athletic equipment, and, yes, changing the rules and style of play of the games we love to watch, as well as the way we teach youngsters how to play them. Additionally, we need to ensure that coaches are educated to use the latest and safest training techniques to reduce the incidence of youth injury in the first place. Unfortunately, resistance to this kind of cultural change is the very thing that may prevent legislation from being truly effective, no matter how many concussion laws are passed in the future.

Of the myriad concerns people have over the push for state and federal concussion legislation, perhaps three issues are the most pressing:

> 1. *Liability.* By making the removal of concussed athletes from play a *legal* issue, some lawmakers (as well as school officials and coaches) have expressed concern that concussion legislation would open a Pandora's box of civil suits. And, indeed, it's a tricky issue. If an athlete lies about concussion symptoms, for example, and is prematurely returned to play, should his coach or school be held legally responsible, to the tune of millions of dollars? It's precisely this question that delayed the Idaho House State Affairs Committee from voting on proposed concussion legislation until consulting with the state attorney general. And though Idaho did eventually pass a concussion law, it is a much weaker bill than the Lystedt model: coaches are not required to remove concussed athletes from games, nor are concussed athletes required to receive written medical clearance before returning to play.[24, 25]
>
> In response to concerns such as these, some states have added specific liability language to concussion legislation. Arizona's Senate Bill 1521, for example, protects from civil litigation doctors who examine concussed athletes, except in cases of gross negligence. Other states, however, may be re-

luctant to pass any laws at all, for fear of an increase in liability suits.

2. *Funding.* Some states, in addition to bolstering return-to-play guidelines, have sought to make preseason baseline testing mandatory for student athletes. Though that's an excellent step in preventing concussed athletes from returning to sports too soon, resolutions such as these require funding to implement—an especially tough challenge for schools that are already strapped for cash. The original proposed federal CONTACT bill (which failed to pass the Senate during the 2010 legislative session) would have taken steps to address the issue of funding, in part by setting aside $5 million for neurocognitive testing and concussion-management programs in its first year of implementation. For now, however, the financial burden sits largely on individual schools and school districts around the nation.

3. *Education.* Athletes, coaches, and athletic trainers from the professional sports world have all expressed concern that the NFL's stricter return-to-play guidelines will actually backfire; that guaranteed time on the bench will only encourage sports stars to hide the symptoms of concussion. "Now that these new guidelines are in place," Hines Ward, wide receiver for the Pittsburgh Steelers (and *Dancing with the Stars* champion), said in an interview with *GQ* magazine, "you'll see more and more guys lying to doctors to stay on the field. Contracts aren't guaranteed. If a guy's contract is coming up and he gets his bell rung . . . trust me, he ain't tellin' nobody."[21] Of course, multimillion-dollar contracts obviously aren't at stake for amateur players, but that same attitude—the propensity to lie about or underplay an injury —is echoed by young athletes across the country. And on some teams, that kind of machismo is even cultivated.

One way to counter this kind of risk is through edu-

Did You Know . . . ?

Although a number of contact sports do not require helmet use, there has been growing controversy over whether certain sports—particularly soccer and women's lacrosse—should mandate helmet use, especially because women seem to be more vulnerable to concussion. But the research is still unclear about whether helmets would reduce the risk, and some experts argue that using helmets in a game where body checking is not allowed may actually *increase* the risk of injury. In a February 2011 article in the *New York Times*, Margot Putukian, MD, director of athletic medicine at Princeton University and chair of the US Lacrosse Sports Science and Safety Committee, explained, "It's hard to absolutely prove, but what we've seen is that behavior can change when athletes feel more protected, especially when it comes to the head and helmets . . . [Athletes] tend to put their bodies and heads in danger that they wouldn't without the protection. And they aren't as protected as they might think."[26]

cation. After all, kids who *understand* the real long-term dangers of concussion, and who know the signs and symptoms, are more likely to be honest about their injuries. Kids who understand concussions are also more likely to watch out for each other. The New Mexico concussion law, for example, one of the country's toughest, has attempted to address what experts call the "code of silence" by encouraging concussions to be reported not only by the injured athletes themselves, but by fellow teammates, too. (Both Preston Plevretes and Ryne Dougherty—two victims of sis—confided in teammates about their symptoms, but hid those symptoms from their doctors.) Yet the educational components of concussion laws vary widely from state to state. In Alabama, for example, school athletes and their parents are required to sign a concussion and head injury information

Did You Know . . . ?

More than thirty states now require concussed student athletes to receive written medical clearance before returning to play. Some legislation, including Washington State's first-of-its-kind Zackery Lystedt Law, mandates that such clearance be provided by a licensed health care professional with training and expertise in concussion. Other states, however, require that the return-to-play decision be made by a "physician."

Here's the problem: neuropsychologists are typically PhDs (as opposed to MDs), so they may not always be considered physicians by law in some states, even though they typically have more expertise than MDs in brain-behavior relationships, traumatic brain injury, concussion management, and neurocognitive testing. If your state requires written medical clearance by a physician, try to consult a neuropsychologist, too. And if you're advocating for a concussion law in your own state, it's important to remember that neuropsychologists should be included in the wording for return-to-play clearance.

sheet each year. In Connecticut, coaches and athletic trainers are required to undergo concussion-management training, but no parental consent to participate in school sports is required. And some state laws don't have any kind of educational component at all.

What all of this means is that no matter how many concussion laws are passed in the future, or how tough those laws may claim to be, the prevention and management of brain injuries really starts at home. It's up to *parents* to make sure that their children understand the risks of brain injury and know the signs and symptoms. It's up to *parents* to instill the notion that lying about concussions or playing through the pain isn't brave, or tough, or cool. It's up to *parents* to change the culture of youth sports, so that our children can enjoy long, safe, and healthy athletic careers. It's up to *parents* to change the game.

WHAT PARENTS CAN DO

One man who is working to change the game is Bobby Hosea. The former pro football player, longtime actor (you might recognize him from guest appearances on *CSI: Crime Scene Investigation* or *24*), well-respected coach, and father of two has made it his mission to protect young football stars by teaching one important skill: tackle with your head *up* instead of *down*.[27]

In the world of football, teaching a youngster to "lead with the head" might be a surefire way to wind up in an emergency room. But that doesn't mean leading with the head isn't happening all the time. Many youth athletic coaches have minimal training or experience to draw from, relying instead on what they were taught about football many years before—perhaps that's why YouTube is chock-full of videos that glorify "monster" tackles and helmet-to-helmet hits among amateur and youth players. Log on, and you'll find clip after clip of kids as young as six getting "laid out," "lit up," or "knocked out," and often at the prodding of a father-coach.

Christopher Nowinski, a former Harvard defensive tackle and well-known concussion awareness advocate, discussed this strange phenomenon in an interview with Sean Gregory of *Time* magazine. He pulled up one video in particular: "Big Football Hit–Helmet to Helmet," which features two eight-year-olds running toward each other, each with his helmet down, until their heads collide with a horrifying crunch. "Who the hell is teaching this?" Nowinski wondered aloud.[22]

Unfortunately, lots of children may be at risk for injuries when put in the hands of ill-informed (if well-intentioned) coaches. Hosea's one-of-a-kind method, on the other hand, which has earned him the reputation of foremost authority on injury preventive tackling, is entirely focused on teaching kids how to avoid headfirst collisions. His Train 'Em Up Academy, a 501(c)3 not-for-profit corporation, was founded not just to protect youth athletes, but also to bring Hosea's method to youth coaches nationwide, by offering coaches clinics and tackling safety certifications.

(Read more about these, as well as Hosea's Take-A-L.A.P. [Learn–Avoid–Prevent] Injury Preventive Fundraiser, at trainemupacademy.org; see also momsteam.com.) But Hosea is also serious about encouraging parents—specifically mothers—to get involved. His academy hosts Moms Tackling Safety Awareness Summits to help mothers learn exactly what causes football-related concussions, and to improve their children's safety.

Hosea isn't the only coach taking steps to change the culture of youth football, to adjust the way the game is played from the inside out. Nor is football the only sport that needs retooling to prevent the prevalence of brain injuries. But Hosea's methods show that it is possible to make organized athletics safer for our children without threatening the integrity, passion, or fun of their chosen sport. Parents need to make sure that their children are joining teams that promote not only safety, but also healthy, positive environments. Coaches should be trained in identifying and managing concussions, but also in how to *teach* their sport in the safest, most effective way. And if your child's coach seems reluctant to adjust his or her style of play, or to take concussion prevention seriously, consider enrolling in a different youth athletic league. Before your child sets foot on an athletic field, ask yourself these questions:

· Are the adults involved in your child's athletic program—the coaches, athletic trainers, and fellow parents—serious about safety? Do they foster a positive athletic environment? Parents and coaches set the tone for a child's athletic experience, so it's important not only to be trained in preventing and managing concussions and other injuries, but also to be respectful and supportive of all the kids on the team. Parents and coaches should never be overly invested in winning, should not tolerate or engage in emotional outbursts or displays of anger, and should never put kids down. Likewise, concussed athletes should never be made to feel as though they are "wimps" or "sissies," and should never suffer negative consequences (such as getting kicked off the team) for taking time off from a sport to fully heal from an injury.

· Is your child confident about his or her athletic abilities, and well suited to play the chosen sport? Watch for signs that your child might be suffering from a lack of confidence on the athletic field. Tossed-off or casual remarks—"I'm not as good as the other players," or "I'll never be good at this game"—might not seem like a big deal, but they are a sign that your child is trying to communicate something to you. So resist the urge to ignore these kinds of statements, and concentrate instead on why your child is feeling this way.

Lack of confidence in sports could signal that your child needs additional training or better-fitting equipment; has an unidentified injury that is hampering her play; is not well suited to the chosen sport (but may excel at something else!); or doesn't enjoy the sport, but continues playing to avoid disappointing the coach, fellow teammates, or maybe even you. Very often, simply lending an ear will do the trick. Listening to your child in a supportive, nonjudgmental way may be just what's needed to give her confidence a boost.

· Is your child's involvement in a particular sport more important to him or to *you*? Sports are an excellent outlet for children to learn independence and gain self-esteem, but youth athletics are also supposed to be *fun*. Adults need to be careful not to put too much pressure on their kids to win at all costs, or to play a sport that they may not be well suited for. Just because Dad was a high school quarterback or Mom was a basketball star doesn't mean that their children will follow suit. Kids need to feel a sense of personal investment in their sport of choice, and the adults in their lives need to put the child's needs first, rather than worry about securing a team's winning record.

Did You Know . . . ?

According to a recent survey by Safe Kids USA, 67 percent of parents "don't worry that much" about sports-related concussions. Even more surprising, 86 percent of the parents polled consider sports-related injuries "just part of the game." Only 9 percent of fathers and 17 percent of mothers think that sports-related injuries can really be prevented.[28]

THE IMPORTANCE OF BRAIN HYGIENE

Just as we make sure our children get their teeth cleaned regularly and undergo routine physical exams, we can take steps to protect their most vital organ—the brain—*before* an injury occurs. Remember: concussions aren't just dings to the head; they're more serious than just "getting your bell rung." And ignoring the signs and symptoms won't make them go away. Always practice brain hygiene, and teach your children to love their brains.

The Ten Principles of Brain Hygiene[29]

1. We each have only one brain; we must care for it and protect it so that it will stay healthy for years to come. The healthier our brains, the longer our athletic careers.
2. Medical or preventive care of our brains is no less important than preseason physicals or properly fitted and reconditioned athletic equipment.
3. Youth athletic personnel, school officials, coaches, parents, and youth athletes should be educated about concussion identification, risk, and management. Learn the signs and symptoms of brain injury.
4. All youth athletes should undergo routine preseason baseline testing.
5. When an athlete is suspected of having sustained a concussion, he or she should be removed from play immediately.

No athlete who exhibits symptoms of concussion should ever be allowed back onto the field. When in doubt, sit them out.

6. Ask any and all health care professionals if they are up to date on the latest concussion identification, treatment, and management guidelines.

7. If you suspect a concussion, seek immediate medical attention.

8. Remember: rest is best for recovery. Limiting mental and physical exertion allows the brain time to heal. No exercise or athletics, no going to the mall, no class trips, no parties, no Facebook or video games, no text messaging, no intense, visually stimulating television, and no reading until physical symptoms begin to subside. Symptomatic children may need a few days off from school, and may need academic accommodations upon return (such as the reduction or elimination of homework and the canceling or postponement of tests) to reduce mental exertion during the early recovery period.

9. The decision to return to play should be made using a team approach. All young athletes should receive three stages of clearance before returning to their sport: (1) medical, (2) neurocognitive, and (3) physical exertional.

10. Concussions in children are different from concussions sustained by adult athletes. Err on the side of caution—extra mental and physical rest and extra time out from athletics—when managing young athletes.

Appendixes

APPENDIX A

Resources

Where to find me:
Rosemarie Scolaro Moser, PHD, ABN, ABPP-RP
Director
Sports Concussion Center of New Jersey at RSM Psychology Center, LLC
3131 Princeton Pike, Building 5
Lawrenceville, NJ 08648
Phone: 609.895.1076
Fax: 609.896.2030
Email: info@sccnj.com
www.sportsconcussionnj.com or www.sccnj.com
www.rsmpsychology.com

Where to learn more about sports concussion:

US Centers for Disease Control and Prevention, www.cdc.gov
The CDC website has the most up-to-date resources on sports concussion, including fact sheets and free tools for coaches, athletes, parents, and health care professionals. You can also view and order concussion posters for youth locker rooms.

MomsTeam, www.momsteam.com
Founded in 2000 by Brooke de Lench (author of *Home Team Advantage: The Critical Role of Mothers in Youth Sports*), MomsTeam is an excellent resource for parents of young athletes. Log on to learn more about concussion identification and management, get updates on the latest concussion legislation, and network with other parents in your area.

Where to find a neuropsychologist in your area:

National Academy of Neuropsychology, www.nanonline.org (click "Online Directory")

Also, most state psychological associations have a referral service that can offer you names of neuropsychologists in your local area.

Where to learn more about baseline and post-concussion test products:

Here are three of the most popular, listed alphabetically:

Axon (formerly CogSport), www.axonsports.com

HeadMinder, www.headminder.com

Impact, www.impacttest.com

Where to find additional information:

· Acute Concussion Evaluation (ACE) form; available in various versions (one for physicians, for example, and one for use at schools)
www.cdc.gov/concussion

· Brain Injury Alliance of New Jersey
www.sportsconcussion.com

· Bobby Hosea's Train 'Em Up Academy tackling camps, coaches' clinics, and Moms Tackling Safety Awareness Summits
www.trainemupacademy.org

· Rep. Bill Pascrell Jr., the Congressional Brain Injury Task Force, and the Concussion Treatment and Care Tools Act (ConTACT)
www.pascrell.house.gov

· Dr. Bennet Omalu and the Brain Injury Research Institute
www.braininjuryresearchinstitute.org

· Center for the Study of Traumatic Encephalopathy and NFL "brain bank"
www.bu.edu/cste

· Hockey Equipment Certification Council Inc.
www.hecc.net

RESOURCES

- National Athletic Trainers' Association
  www.nata.org
- National Operating Committee on Standards for Athletic
  Equipment
  www.nocsae.org
- Sports Legacy Institute
  www.sportslegacy.org
- Virginia Tech National Impact Database helmet safety research
  www.sbes.vt.edu/nid.php

APPENDIX B

Test Your Concussion Knowledge: Answers

1. *False.* Each concussion is unique, and the severity of a concussion cannot actually be determined until *after* the athlete has fully recovered. In fact, only about 10 percent of concussed athletes ever "black out."[1] It's not uncommon for an athlete who lost consciousness to recover more quickly than one who demonstrated less visible, immediate symptoms, but suffered from a persistent headache for months.

2. *False.* In football (and most other contact sports), the job of the helmet is to protect against *focal* injuries, which may affect discrete, specific parts of the brain as a result of impact. For example, skull fractures and hemorrhages (bleeding in the brain) are types of focal injuries. You can think about it this way: in a high-speed car accident, a passenger's head might slam into the windshield, shattering the skull and resulting in swelling and bleeding of the brain. A concussion, on the other hand, is defined as the brief neurological impairment (including confusion, headache, amnesia, or loss of consciousness) that results from impact or a strong force, so it may not be caused by a direct hit to the head; a blow to the body or a whiplash motion can cause the brain to slam against the *inside* of the skull. No helmet can protect against or prevent that.

3. *False.* Young women are more susceptible than young men to concussion.[2] Though there are several theories about the reason, none has been proven yet. You can read more about girls' vulnerability to concussion in Chapter 1.

4. *False.* Sideline assessment tests are useful to *document* the immediate signs of a concussion, but by themselves they are not diagnostic, nor can they determine the severity of a concussion. It doesn't matter how "well" your child performs on a sideline

assessment test; we still won't know the severity of the injury until *after* he or she has fully recovered.

5. *False.* Children often don't exhibit any symptoms of concussion until *days* after a hit or tackle. If you suspect that your child has sustained a concussion, he or she must be removed from play immediately, and should not return until undergoing a medical exam; submitting to post-concussion neurocognitive testing; completing a course of mental and physical rest; undergoing physical exertional testing and a graduated reconditioning; and then receiving formal clearance to return to the field from a pediatrician, physician, neuropsychologist, or other licensed health care professional. State laws may dictate exactly which type of health care professional may provide this formal clearance.

6. *False.* CT scans and MRIS aren't sensitive enough to detect biochemical changes in the brain that result from concussion. Rather, these tests are used to detect focal injuries and *gross pathology*, such as a hemorrhage or brain bleed. The vast majority of concussions will not show up on a routine CT scan or MRI.

7. *False.* At this time, the majority of general physicians, pediatricians, ER doctors, and even some neurologists in the United States are not up to date on concussion management and treatment, especially in children. While the state of concussion management is changing rapidly—particularly with the introduction of state laws that seek to standardize treatment—it is still not uncommon to find that some parents of concussed children are more up to date on treatment and recovery than are the health care professionals to whom they have been referred.

8. *True.* In my experience, most concussions in children take *more than* a week or two to resolve, and that's assuming the child was put on adequate rest, did not return to play, and did not overexert himself or herself during recovery. High school athletes, in particular, tend to show a dip in cognitive ability around day eight following a concussive blow.[3] Research indicates that children who do not get adequate mental and physical rest after a concussion may exhibit symptoms for an even longer period of time.[4]

9. *False.* The "three strikes and you're out" rule has little to no research basis. It's also not a particularly helpful or informed position. Each athlete's history of concussion is different; a child who
   sustained three concussions over a period of ten years, with three
   or more years between incidents, is not the same as a child whose
   concussions occurred in a single calendar year.

10. *True.* A history of undiagnosed concussions can cause symptoms
    including difficulty concentrating, fatigue, memory problems,
    impulsivity, temper outbursts, and a low frustration threshold,
    all of which are also hallmarks of ADHD. I've had a number of
    adolescents referred to me for neuropsychological evaluations to
    test for possible learning, attention, or behavioral disorders, only
    to discover that the culprit is actually head trauma. You can read
    more about the commonalities between post-concussion syn-
    drome and ADHD in Chapter 2.

APPENDIX C

The Sports Concussion Center of New Jersey
Sports Concussion Card
www.SportsConcussionNJ.com

POSSIBLE SIGNS & SYMPTOMS	IF YOU SUSPECT A CONCUSSION	TIPS TO REMEMBER
· Dizziness · Confusion · Headache · Fatique · Nausea or Vomiting · Feeling "dazed" or "foggy" · Balance problems · Blurred or double vision · Blacking out or loss of consciousness · Amnesia or trouble remembering · Numbness or tingling · Changes in emotional status or behavior · Feeling like your child "just isn't right"	#1. Immediately remove the athlete from play #2. Have the athlete evaluated by a licensed health care professional with expertise in concussion identification and management #3. Star the athlete on a course of mental and physical rest until symptom-free #4. Avoid sports and athletic activity until the athlete is cleared to return to play #5. Abide by concussion laws and guidelines in your state, city or school district #6. When in doubt, sit them out!	You don't have to hit your head to sustain a concussion. The presence of any single symptom is enough to suspect a brain injury Helmets and mouth guards can not completely prevent concussions. Symptoms of a brain injury may not appear until days after a hard hit or rough tackle. Neuroimaging tests (CT scans or MRIs) are usually "normal" after a concussion. Sustaining a second hit before fully recovering from the first may cause Second Impact Syndrome, an often fatal condition. *REST IS BEST* for a full, speedy recovery. Always be safe, and always practice Brain Hygiene.

The information presented here is not a substitute for medical diagnosis or treatment by a licensed health professional.

The Academic Phases of Concussion Recovery

Youth athletes who have sustained a concussion generally fall into the following categories or *phases* of recovery, depending on the severity and course of healing. A neuropsychologist can help the school tailor a program and timeline of academic accommodations to fit the needs and recovery course of the athlete.

1. Acute Phase

In the days and weeks following a concussion, it is critical that youth get as much mental and physical rest as possible until symptoms begin to subside.

Comprehensive rest means:

- · No text messaging
- · No video games
- · No computer use
- · No school, homework, or tests
- · No reading
- · No parties, dances, trips, or social outings
- · Extremely limited access to television
- · No physical exertion, exercise, or working up a sweat

2. Recovery Phase

As an athlete's symptoms subside and his post-concussion neurocognitive test scores return to baseline or have stabilized, he can begin returning to his daily routine. It's important to move slowly, however, introducing activities carefully so that headaches and other symptoms do not return.

· Start with partial school days and then transition to full days with frequent rest breaks.

· Start by avoiding note-taking, homework, and tests, then transition slowly to completing assignments on extended deadlines.

· Look for alternative ways to complete assignments. For example, employ audiobooks instead of reading printed matter, consider oral instead of written exams, use modified short quizzes or papers instead of long midterms, or allow the student to makeup missed assignments during vacation or school breaks.

· Make sure your child is excused from gym class until he has been medically cleared to begin noncontact exercise.

3. Chronic Phase

Sometimes, a youth athlete may experience more long lasting or chronic symptoms that significantly limit her ability to concentrate, focus, study, and learn. In such cases, one or more of the following actions may be implemented by the school district:

· A 504 Plan, which documents the academic accommodations requested.

· Individualized Education Plan (IEP), which involves the formal classification of a student's difficulties so that a comprehensive plan of academic accommodations and special education programming can be put into place.

· Home schooling, which allows the student to maximize rest time and condense academic time so as not to fall behind.

· Medical leave of absence, which may be needed if the student's symptoms are so severe that academics cannot be successfully completed and more comprehensive rest is required.

State-by-State Guide to New and Pending Concussion Legislation

Does your state have a concussion law in place?

In 2009, Washington became the first state to pass strict and sweeping concussion legislation, aimed at protecting children from the long-term effects of sports-related brain injuries and preventing injured student athletes from returning to play too soon. Since then, thirty-three states have passed similar bills (at the time of this writing, another ten states have legislation pending).

Although the scope of each law varies from state to state, the first-of-its-kind Washington State bill—informally known as the Zackery Lystedt Law—has served as a model for a majority of legislators. Bills that contain all three of the Lystedt law's principal tenets—(1) concussion awareness and education, (2) mandatory removal from play, and (3) written medical clearance before returning to play—are generally considered strong laws. (Conversely, bills that do not contain all three tenets are considered weak and, therefore, less effective.)

Find out if your state has a concussion law in place, if parents are required to provide written consent before children are allowed to participate in school sports, and if concussion laws in your area extend to community-based or recreational athletic leagues. For updated information, log on to www.momsteam .com.

Alabama

HOUSE BILL 108
SIGNED INTO LAW: JUNE 2011
EFFECTIVE: IMMEDIATELY UPON PASSAGE

Education: Calls for the governing body of each sport or recreational organization to develop concussion-management guidelines. Coaches must receive
annual training in concussion identification and management.
Mandatory parental consent: Yes. Youth athletes and a parent or guardian must
sign a concussion and head injury information sheet on a yearly basis.

Immediate removal from play: Yes. Any athlete suspected of having sustained a concussion in a practice or game must be immediately removed from play and is barred from same-day return to play.

Return-to-play guidelines and clearance: Concussed athletes must be evaluated by and receive written consent from a licensed physician before returning to play.

Application to private leagues: Yes. Extends to youth and recreation leagues.

Alaska

HOUSE BILL 15

SIGNED INTO LAW: MAY 2011

EFFECTIVE: START OF THE 2011–2012 SCHOOL YEAR

Education: Calls for the governing body of the school district to consult with the Alaska School Activities Association to develop concussion-management guidelines.

Mandatory parental consent: No

Immediate removal from play: Yes. Any athlete suspected of having sustained a concussion in a practice or game must be immediately removed from play and is barred from same-day return to play.

Return-to-play guidelines and clearance: Concussed athletes must be evaluated by and receive written consent from a licensed health care provider with specific training in the evaluation and management of concussion before returning to play.

Application to private leagues: None

Arizona

SENATE BILL 1521

SIGNED INTO LAW: APRIL 2011

EFFECTIVE: JULY 2011

Education: Calls for individual school districts to develop guidelines and educational programs.

Mandatory parental consent: Yes. Youth athletes and a parent or guardian must sign a concussion and head injury information sheet on a yearly basis.

Immediate removal from play: Yes. Any athlete suspected of having sustained a concussion in a practice or game must be immediately removed from play and is barred from same-day return to play. If a licensed health care provider rules out a concussion at the time of injury, however, a student may return to play on the same day.

Return-to-play guidelines and clearance: Concussed athletes must be evaluated by and receive written consent from a licensed health care provider (specifically, a physician, athletic trainer, nurse practitioner, or physician assistant) with training in the evaluation and management of concussion before returning to play.

Application to private leagues: Only those private community-based or recreational leagues that are operating on school or school-district owned or operated facilities are subject to the concussion-management law.

Arkansas

No concussion legislation is pending at this time.

California

ASSEMBLY BILL 25
SIGNED INTO LAW: OCTOBER 2011
EFFECTIVE: IMMEDIATELY UPON PASSAGE

Education: No

Mandatory parental consent: Yes. Youth athletes and a parent or guardian must sign a concussion and head injury information sheet on a yearly basis.

Immediate removal from play: Yes. Any athlete suspected of having sustained a concussion in a practice or game must be immediately removed from play and is barred from same-day return to play.

Return-to-play guidelines and clearance: Concussed athletes must be evaluated by and receive written consent from a licensed health care provider with specific training in the evaluation and management of concussion before returning to play.

Application to private leagues: Yes. Youth sports and recreation programs must provide a statement of compliance with concussion-management guidelines to the governing board of a school district before using any public school facility.

Colorado

SENATE BILL 40: JAKE SNAKENBERG YOUTH CONCUSSION ACT

NAMED IN HONOR OF JAKE SNAKENBERG, A HIGH SCHOOL FOOTBALL PLAYER
  WHO DEVELOPED SECOND IMPACT SYNDROME AND DIED IN 2004

SIGNED INTO LAW: MARCH 2011

EFFECTIVE: JANUARY 2012

Education: Coaches (including coaches of youth athletic leagues) must receive annual training in concussion identification and management.

Mandatory parental consent: No

Immediate removal from play: Yes. Any athlete suspected of having sustained a concussion in a practice or game must be immediately removed from play.

Return-to-play guidelines and clearance: Concussed athletes, if their symptoms cannot be "readily explained by a condition other than concussion," must be evaluated by and receive written consent from a licensed health care provider (specifically, a doctor of medicine, doctor of osteopathic medicine, nurse practitioner, physician assistant, or doctor of psychology with training in neuropsychogy) before returning to play. Additionally, the athlete's parents must be notified.

Application to private leagues: Yes. Extends to youth and recreation leagues, as well as public and nonpublic middle, junior high, and high schools. Colorado is one of the few states that extend coverage to athletes below middle school (the law applies to children ages eleven to nineteen).

Connecticut

SENATE BILL 456

SIGNED INTO LAW: MAY 2010

EFFECTIVE: JULY 2010

Education: Coaches are required to take an initial training course regarding the identification and management of concussions and head injuries, as well as yearly refresher courses.

Mandatory parental consent: No

Immediate removal from play: Yes. Any athlete suspected of having sustained a concussion in a practice or game must be immediately removed from play and is barred from same-day return to play.

Return-to-play guidelines and clearance: Concussed athletes must be evaluated by and receive written consent from a licensed health care provider (specifically, a physician, physician assistant, advanced practice registered nurse, or athletic trainer) with training in the evaluation and management of concussion before returning to play. Additionally, the athlete must no longer be experiencing any symptoms of concussion.

Application to private leagues: None

Penalties: Coaches in violation of this law may have their coaching permits revoked by the board of education.

Delaware

SENATE BILL 111

SIGNED INTO LAW: AUGUST 2011

EFFECTIVE: NO LATER THAN THE 2012–2013 SCHOOL YEAR

Education: Calls for the Delaware Interscholastic Athletic Association (DIAA) to adopt regulations regarding the appropriate recognition and management of concussions. Requires coaches to complete concussion training consistent with DIAA regulations.

Mandatory parental consent: Yes. Youth athletes and a parent or guardian must sign a concussion and head injury information sheet on a yearly basis.

Immediate removal from play: Yes. Any athlete suspected of having sustained a concussion in a practice or game must be immediately removed from play.

Return-to-play guidelines and clearance: Concussed athletes must receive medical assessment or clearance before returning to play, in accordance with DIAA regulations.

Application to private leagues: None

District of Columbia

BILL 19–7

SIGNED INTO LAW: JULY 2011

EFFECTIVE: THIRTY DAYS AFTER PASSAGE

Education: Calls for the mayor to establish a concussion training program, and to determine which individuals should be made to complete such a program.

Mandatory parental consent: Yes. Youth athletes and a parent or guardian must sign a statement acknowledging receipt of concussion-related educational materials.

Immediate removal from play: Yes. Any athlete suspected of having sustained a concussion in a practice or game must be immediately removed from play.

Return-to-play guidelines and clearance: Concussed athletes must be evaluated by and receive written consent from a licensed health care provider before returning to play.

Application to private leagues: Extends to all athletes under age eighteen who participate in athletic programs operated by public, nonpublic, charter, or parochial schools, by the department of parks and recreation, or by any nonprofit or for-profit organization, as well as youth athletes participating in physical education class.

Florida

HOUSE BILL 301

SENATE BILL 730

Status: Pending. The bill did not pass during the 2011 legislative session.

Georgia

HOUSE BILL 673

Status: Pending.

Hawaii

HOUSE BILL 622 AND OTHERS

Status: Pending

Idaho

HOUSE BILL 676
SIGNED INTO LAW: APRIL 2011
EFFECTIVE: START OF THE 2011–2012 SCHOOL YEAR

Education: Calls for the state board of education to collaborate with the Idaho High School Activities Association to develop guidelines and educational materials to inform parents, coaches, and athletes about the dangers and risk of concussion.
Mandatory parental consent: No
Immediate removal from play: No
Return-to-play guidelines and clearance: None
Application to private leagues: None

Illinois

HOUSE BILL 200
SIGNED INTO LAW: JULY 2011
EFFECTIVE: IMMEDIATELY

Education: Calls for school boards to establish a concussion policy that complies with the protocols of the Illinois High School Association.
Mandatory parental consent: Yes. Youth athletes and a parent or guardian must sign a concussion and head injury information sheet on a yearly basis.
Immediate removal from play: Yes. Any athlete suspected of having sustained a concussion in a practice or game must be immediately removed from play.
Return-to-play guidelines and clearance: Concussed athletes must be evaluated by and receive written consent from a licensed health care provider before returning to play.
Application to private leagues: None

Indiana

SENATE BILL 93

SIGNED INTO LAW: MAY 2011

EFFECTIVE: JULY 2011

Education: Calls for the department of education to develop and disseminate concussion guidelines and information sheets.

Mandatory parental consent: Yes. Youth athletes and a parent or guardian must sign a concussion and head injury information sheet on a yearly basis.

Immediate removal from play: Yes. Any athlete suspected of having sustained a concussion in a practice or game must be immediately removed from play.

Return-to-play guidelines and clearance: Concussed athletes must be evaluated by and receive written consent from a licensed health care provider with specific training in the evaluation and management of concussion before returning to play.

Application to private leagues: None

Iowa

HOUSE FILE 581

SENATE FILE 267

SIGNED INTO LAW: APRIL 2011

EFFECTIVE: JULY 2011

Education: Calls on the Iowa High School Athletic Association and the Iowa Girls High School Athletic Union to work together in distributing concussion-management guidelines based on information from the US Centers for Disease Control and Prevention.

Mandatory parental consent: Yes. Youth athletes and a parent or guardian must sign a concussion and head injury information sheet on a yearly basis.

Immediate removal from play: Yes. Any athlete suspected of having sustained a concussion in a practice or game must be immediately removed from play.

Return-to-play guidelines and clearance: Concussed athletes must be evaluated by and receive written consent from a licensed health care provider (specifically, a physician, physician assistant, chiropractor, advanced registered nurse practitioner, nurse, physical therapist, or athletic trainer) with specific training in the evaluation and management of concussion before returning to play.

Application to private leagues: None. But it does apply to both public and non-public schools, grades 7–12, as well as any and all interscholastic activities, contests, and practices.

Kansas

SENATE BILL 33
SIGNED INTO LAW: MAY 2011
EFFECTIVE: IMMEDIATELY

Education: Calls for the board of education, in cooperation with the Kansas High School Activities Association, to compile and distribute information on concussion to coaches, athletes, and parents.

Mandatory parental consent: Yes. Youth athletes and a parent or guardian must sign a concussion and head injury information sheet on a yearly basis.

Immediate removal from play: Yes. Any athlete suspected of having sustained a concussion in a practice or game must be immediately removed from play.

Return-to-play guidelines and clearance: Concussed athletes must be evaluated by and receive written consent from a licensed health care provider before returning to play.

Application to private leagues: None. But it does include all public and accredited nonpublic high schools, middle schools, and junior high schools.

Kentucky

HOUSE RESOLUTION 58

Status: Pending.

Louisiana

SENATE BILL 189
SIGNED INTO LAW: JUNE 2011
EFFECTIVE: IMMEDIATELY

Education: Calls for the Louisiana Department of Health and Hospitals to develop concussion-management guidelines. All coaches and officials must complete concussion identification and management training annually.

Mandatory parental consent: Yes. Youth athletes and a parent or guardian must sign a concussion and head injury information sheet on a yearly basis.

Immediate removal from play: Yes. Any athlete suspected of having sustained a concussion in a practice or game must be immediately removed from play.

Return-to-play guidelines and clearance: Concussed athletes, if their symptoms cannot be "readily explained by a condition other than concussion," must be evaluated by and receive written consent from a licensed health care provider (specifically, a physician, licensed nurse practitioner, physician assistant, or psychologist with training in neuropsychology) before returning to play. Additionally, the athlete's parents must be notified.

Application to private leagues: Yes. Extends to all public and nonpublic elementary, middle, junior high, and high schools, as well as all private and recreational athletic clubs and leagues, where the majority of participants are age seven years or older, and under age nineteen.

Maine

LEGISLATIVE DOCUMENT 98

Status: Pending

Maryland

SENATE BILL 771
HOUSE BILL 858
SIGNED INTO LAW: MAY 2011
EFFECTIVE: JULY 2011

Education: Calls for the department of education to collaborate with multiple organizations (including the Maryland Department of Health and Mental Hygiene, the Maryland Public Secondary Schools Athletic Association, and the Brain Injury Association of Maryland), to develop concussion-management guidelines.

Mandatory parental consent: Yes. Youth athletes and a parent or guardian must sign a concussion and head injury information sheet on a yearly basis.

Immediate removal from play: Yes. Any athlete suspected of having sustained a concussion in a practice or game must be immediately removed from play.

Return-to-play guidelines and clearance: Concussed athletes must be evaluated by and receive written consent from a licensed health care provider with specific training in the evaluation and management of concussion before returning to play.

Application to private leagues: Yes. Extends to athletes age seventeen and under who participate in school-sponsored or recreational athletic organizations, as well as individuals of any age who are physically or mentally handicapped and participate in an athletic league. Youth sports programs must provide the county board a statement of compliance with concussion-management guidelines before using any public school facility.

Massachusetts

SENATE BILL 2469

SIGNED INTO LAW: JULY 2010

EFFECTIVE: JULY 2010

Education: Calls for the development of an interscholastic athletic head injury safety training program. Annual participation in the program is required by coaches, athletic trainers, parent volunteers, school athletic directors, directors of school marching bands, physicians and nurses employed by a school or school district or who volunteer to assist with any extracurricular athletic activity, as well as a *parent or guardian of children participating in extracurricular athletic activity*. Additionally, coaches, athletic trainers, and volunteers are not permitted to encourage "dangerous" athletic technique or activity, including using a helmet or other sports equipment as a "weapon."

Mandatory parental consent: Yes. Youth athletes and a parent or guardian must sign a statement acknowledging receipt of concussion-related educational materials. Additionally, student athletes must provide information about any previous sports-related head injury at the start of each season.

Immediate removal from play: Yes. Any athlete suspected of having sustained a concussion in a practice or game, or any athlete who loses consciousness during a practice or game, must be immediately removed from play.

Return-to-play guidelines and clearance: Concussed athletes must be evaluated by and receive written consent from a licensed health care provider (specifically, a physician, neuropsychologist, athletic trainer, or some other appropriately trained or licensed health care provider as determined by the department of public health) before returning to play.

Application to private leagues: None. Applies to public and nonpublic schools only.

Michigan

HOUSE BILL 4396

Status: Pending

Minnesota

HOUSE FILE 905

SENATE FILE 612

SIGNED INTO LAW: MAY 2011

EFFECTIVE: SEPTEMBER 2011

Education: Calls for the governing body of each sport to work with the department of education to provide concussion-management guidelines. Coaches and officials are required to complete yearly concussion identification and management training.

Mandatory parental consent: Yes. Youth athletes and a parent or guardian must sign a concussion information form on a yearly basis.

Immediate removal from play: Yes. Any athlete suspected of having sustained a concussion in a practice or game must be immediately removed from play.

Return-to-play guidelines and clearance: Concussed athletes must be evaluated by and receive written consent from a licensed health care provider with specific training in the evaluation and management of concussion before returning to play. Additionally, athletes must no longer be exhibiting symptoms of concussion.

Application to private leagues: Yes. Extends to any city, business, or nonprofit organization that organizes a youth athletic activity and requires a fee to participate or whose cost to participate is sponsored by a business or nonprofit organization.

Mississippi

SENATE BILL 2271

Status: Pending.

Missouri

HOUSE BILL 300
HOUSE BILL 334
HOUSE BILL 387
SIGNED INTO LAW: JULY 2011
EFFECTIVE: AUGUST 2011

Education: Calls for the Missouri Department of Health and Senior Services to work with numerous agencies (including a statewide association of school boards) to develop concussion-management guidelines.
Mandatory parental consent: Yes. Youth athletes and a parent or guardian must sign a concussion and brain injury information sheet on a yearly basis.
Immediate removal from play: Yes. Any athlete suspected of having sustained a concussion in a practice or game must be immediately removed from play and is barred from same day return to play.
Return-to-play guidelines and clearance: Concussed athletes must be evaluated by and receive written consent from a licensed health care provider with specific training in the evaluation and management of concussion before returning to play.
Application to private leagues: None

Montana

No concussion legislation is pending at this time.

Nebraska

LEGISLATIVE BILL 260

SIGNED INTO LAW: APRIL 2011

EFFECTIVE: JULY 2012

Education: Calls for schools and youth athletic leagues to distribute educational materials to student athletes, coaches, and parents. Educational materials must be approved by a chief medical officer or licensed health care provider with training in the identification and management of concussions in the pediatric population.

Mandatory parental consent: No

Immediate removal from play: Yes. Any athlete suspected of having sustained a concussion in a practice or game must be immediately removed from play.

Return-to-play guidelines and clearance: Concussed athletes must be evaluated by and receive written consent from a licensed health care provider (specifically, a physician, certified athletic trainer, neuropsychologist, or some other qualified individual who is recognized by the State of Nebraska to provide health care services and who has been trained in the evaluation and management of concussions) before returning to play. Additionally, the athlete's parents must be notified.

Application to private leagues: Yes. Extends to any city, business, or nonprofit organization that organizes a youth athletic activity for children ages nineteen and younger and requires a fee to participate, or whose cost to participate is sponsored by a business or nonprofit organization.

Nevada

ASSEMBLY BILL 455

Status: Pending

New Hampshire

SENATE BILL 95

Status: Pending

New Jersey

ASSEMBLY BILL 2743

SIGNED INTO LAW: DECEMBER 2010

EFFECTIVE: START OF THE 2011–2012 SCHOOL YEAR

Education: Calls for the department of education, in consultation with the Commissioner of the New Jersey Department of Health and Senior Services, to develop a concussion-management training program, which must be attended by school physicians, public and nonpublic school athletic coaches, and athletic trainers. Athletic trainers are required to complete twenty-four credits of continuing education, which shall include training in the management of concussions, as a condition of license renewal.

Mandatory parental consent: Yes. Youth athletes and a parent or guardian must sign a concussion and brain injury information sheet on a yearly basis.

Immediate removal from play: Yes. Any athlete suspected of having sustained a concussion in a practice or game must be immediately removed from play.

Return-to-play guidelines and clearance: Concussed athletes must be evaluated by a licensed health care provider with specific training in the evaluation and management of concussion, and must receive written consent from a licensed physician with specific training in the evaluation and management of concussion before returning to play.

Application to private leagues: None

New Mexico

SENATE BILL 1

SIGNED INTO LAW: MARCH 2010

EFFECTIVE: AUGUST 2010

Education: Calls for the New Mexico Activities Association to consult with school districts and the New Mexico Brain Injury Advisory Council to develop brain injury management guidelines. Coaches must undergo concussion identification and management training.

Mandatory parental consent: Yes. Youth athletes and a parent or guardian must sign a concussion and brain injury information sheet on a yearly basis.

Immediate removal from play: Yes. Any athlete suspected of having sustained a concussion in a practice or game must be immediately removed from play and is barred from same-day return to play.

Return-to-play guidelines and clearance: Concussed athletes must be evaluated by and receive written consent from a licensed health care provider (specifically, a physician, physician assistant, osteopathic physician, certified nurse practitioner, osteopathic physician assistant, psychologist, or athletic trainer) before returning to play. Additionally, concussed athletes must no longer exhibit symptoms and must wait *a minimum of one week from the date of injury* before returning to play.

Application to private leagues: None. Extends to junior high and high school only.

New York

SENATE BILL 3953-A
SIGNED INTO LAW: SEPTEMBER 2011
EFFECTIVE: JULY 2012

Education: Requires each school district and non-public school to appoint a concussion-management team. Each team will consist of the athletic director (if any), school nurse, school doctor, a coach, an athletic trainer, and other personnel as designated by the school district. Concussion-management teams are responsible for creating a concussion information pamphlet, which must be distributed to student athletes and their parents, as well as physical education teachers and coaches. Concussion-management teams must also enact guidelines for providing academic accommodations to concussed athletes. Additionally, all coaches, physical education teachers, nurses, and athletic trainers must complete concussion training every other year.

Mandatory parental consent: Yes. Youth athletes and a parent or guardian must sign a form indicating receipt of the concussion information pamphlet. This form must be kept on file as part of the student's permanent health record.

Immediate removal from play: Yes. Any athlete suspected of having sustained a concussion in a practice or game must be immediately removed from play and is barred from same-day return to play. Suspected concussions must be reported to the department of health.

Return-to-play guidelines and clearance: Concussed athletes must be evaluated by and receive written consent from a licensed physician with specific training in the evaluation and management of concussion before returning to play. This written medical clearance must be kept on file as part of the student's permanent health record. Additionally, concussed athletes must be symptom-free for a minimum of twenty-four hours before returning to play.

Application to private leagues: None

North Carolina

HOUSE BILL 792: GFELLER-WALLER CONCUSSION AWARENESS ACT

NAMED IN HONOR OF MATT GFELLER AND JAQUAN WALLER, TWO

   HIGH SCHOOL FOOTBALL PLAYERS WHO DIED OF FOOTBALL-RELATED

   CONCUSSION COMPLICATIONS IN 2008

SIGNED INTO LAW: JUNE 2011

EFFECTIVE: IMMEDIATELY

Education: Calls for the Matthew A. Gfeller Sport-Related Traumatic Brain Injury Research Center to work with multiple organizations (including the North Carolina Athletic Trainers' Association and the North Carolina High School Athletic Association) to develop concussion-management guidelines. Schools are also required to develop venue-specific emergency action plan(s) to deal with serious injuries, in which a student athlete's condition may deteriorate rapidly.

Mandatory parental consent: Yes. Youth athletes and a parent or guardian must sign a concussion and head injury information sheet on a yearly basis.

Immediate removal from play: Yes. Any athlete suspected of having sustained a concussion in a practice or game must be immediately removed from play and is barred from same-day return to play.

Return-to-play guidelines and clearance: Concussed athletes must be evaluated by and receive written consent from a licensed health care provider (specifically, a physician, a neuropsychologist working in consultation with a physician, athletic trainer, physician assistant, or nurse practitioner) with training in the evaluation and management of concussion before returning to play.

Application to private leagues: None. Applies only to middle and high schools.

North Dakota

SENATE BILL 2281

SIGNED INTO LAW: APRIL 2011

EFFECTIVE: AUGUST 2011

Education: Mandates that all school-sanctioned athletic activities are subject to a concussion-management program. Coaches, athletic trainers, and officials must complete training about the identification and management of concussions every two years.

Mandatory parental consent: Yes. Youth athletes and a parent or guardian must sign a statement acknowledging receipt of concussion-related educational materials.

Immediate removal from play: Yes. Any athlete suspected of having sustained a concussion in a practice or game must be immediately removed from play.

Return-to-play guidelines and clearance: Concussed athletes must be evaluated by and receive written consent from a licensed health care provider with specific training in the evaluation and management of concussion before returning to play.

Application to private leagues: None. Applies to public and nonpublic schools only.

Ohio

HOUSE BILL 143

Status: Pending

Oklahoma

SENATE BILL 1700
SIGNED INTO LAW: MAY 2010
EFFECTIVE: JULY 2010

Education: Calls for the board of education to work with the Oklahoma Secondary Schools Activities Association to develop concussion guidelines.

Mandatory parental consent: Yes. Youth athletes and a parent or guardian must sign a concussion and head injury information sheet on a yearly basis.

Immediate removal from play: Yes. Any athlete suspected of having sustained a concussion in a practice or game must be immediately removed from play.

Return-to-play guidelines and clearance: Concussed athletes must be evaluated by and receive written consent from a licensed health care provider with specific training in the evaluation and management of concussion before returning to play.

Application to private leagues: None

Oregon

SENATE BILL 348: "MAX'S LAW"
NAMED IN HONOR OF MAX CONRADT, A HIGH SCHOOL FOOTBALL PLAYER
   WHO DEVELOPED SECOND IMPACT SYNDROME IN 2001
SIGNED INTO LAW: JUNE 2009
EFFECTIVE: START OF THE 2010–2011 SCHOOL YEAR

Education: School coaches must receive annual training in concussion identification and management.

Mandatory parental consent: No

Immediate removal from play: Yes. Any athlete suspected of having sustained a concussion in a practice or game must be immediately removed from play and is barred from same-day return to play.

Return-to-play guidelines and clearance: Concussed athletes may return to play no sooner than one day after injury. Additionally, concussed athletes must no longer exhibit symptoms, and must receive written consent from a licensed health care provider.

Application to private leagues: None

Pennsylvania

SENATE BILL 200

SIGNED INTO LAW: NOVEMBER 2011

EFFECTIVE: JULY 2012

Education: Calls for the Pennsylvania departments of public health and education to develop concussion guidelines. Additionally, school coaches must receive annual training in concussion identification and management.

Mandatory parental consent: Yes. Youth athletes and a parent or guardian must sign a concussion and head injury information sheet on a yearly basis.

Immediate removal from play: Yes. Any athlete suspected of having sustained a concussion in a practice or game must be immediately removed from play.

Return-to-play guidelines and clearance: Concussed athletes must be evaluated by and receive written consent from an "appropriate" licensed medical professional (specifically, a physician, a certified health care professional designated by a physician, or a psychologist with training in neuropsychology) with specific training in the evaluation and management of concussion before returning to play.

Application to private leagues: None

Penalties: Public schools are required to establish minimum penalties for any coach who (1) fails to sideline an athlete who is exhibiting the signs or symptoms of a concussion, or (2) allows a concussed athlete to return to play without medical clearance. The first violation will mandate a suspension from coaching for the remainder of the season. The second violation will mandate a suspension from coaching for the remainder of the season and the following season. The third violation will result in permanent suspension from coaching.

Rhode Island

SENATE BILL 2034

SIGNED INTO LAW: JUNE 2010

EFFECTIVE: JULY 2010

In 2011, statewide concussion legislation was expanded with the passage of House Bill 5440A and Senate Bill 0291A.

Education: Calls for the department of education and the department of health to work with the Rhode Island Interscholastic League to develop concussion guidelines. All coaches and volunteers must undergo concussion identification and management training and must attend annual refresher courses. Baseline testing is encouraged but not required.

Mandatory parental consent: Yes. Youth athletes and a parent or guardian must sign a concussion and head injury information sheet on a yearly basis.

Immediate removal from play: Yes. Any athlete suspected of having sustained a concussion in a practice or game must be immediately removed from play.

Return-to-play guidelines and clearance: Concussed athletes must be evaluated by and receive written consent from a licensed physician before returning to play.

Application to private leagues: None

South Carolina

HOUSE BILL 3768

Status: Pending

South Dakota

SENATE BILL 149

SIGNED INTO LAW: MARCH 2011

EFFECTIVE: IMMEDIATELY

Education: The department of education and the South Dakota High School Activities Association must work together to develop concussion-management guidelines. Coaches must undergo concussion identification and management training every year.

Mandatory parental consent: Yes. Youth athletes and a parent or guardian must sign a concussion and head injury information sheet on a yearly basis.

Immediate removal from play: Yes. Any athlete suspected of having sustained a concussion in a practice or game must be immediately removed from play.

Return-to-play guidelines and clearance: Concussed athletes must be evaluated by and receive written consent from a licensed health care provider with specific training in the evaluation and management of concussion before returning to play. Additionally, the concussed athlete must not be exhibiting any symptoms or behaviors of concussion.

Application to private leagues: None

Tennessee

SENATE BILL 1120

SENATE BILL 841

SENATE BILL 589

Status: Pending

Texas

HOUSE BILL 2038: "NATASHA'S LAW"

NAMED IN HONOR OF NATASHA HELMICK, A FORMER HIGH SCHOOL SOCCER
    PLAYER WHO GAVE UP THE GAME AFTER SUFFERING MULTIPLE CONCUSSIONS

SIGNED INTO LAW: JUNE 2011

EFFECTIVE: IMMEDIATELY

Education: In this first-of-its-kind legislation, Texas requires each school district to appoint a concussion oversight team. Each team must include a licensed physician and *at least* one additional member, either an athletic trainer, advanced practice nurse, neuropsychologist, or physician assistant. All team members must have training in the identification and management of concussions and are required to stay up to date in their concussion training. Concussion oversight teams are responsible for establishing return-to-play protocols. Additionally, coaches and athletic trainers must receive concussion training at least every two years.

Mandatory parental consent: Yes. Youth athletes and a parent or guardian must sign a concussion and head injury information sheet on a yearly basis.

Immediate removal from play: Yes. Any athlete suspected of having sustained a concussion in a practice or game must be immediately removed from play.

Return-to-play guidelines and clearance: Concussed athletes must be evaluated by and receive written consent from a licensed physician before returning to play. In addition, concussed athletes and their parents must sign a consent inform indicating that the athlete has abided by the return-to-play protocol (as established by the concussion oversight team), understands the risks associated with returning to play, and understands certain immunity provisions.

Application to private leagues: None

Utah

HOUSE BILL 204
SIGNED INTO LAW: MARCH 2011
EFFECTIVE: MAY 2011

Education: Calls for all amateur sports organizations (including school athletic teams) to adopt and enforce a concussion policy and to inform parents and legal guardians of that policy.

Mandatory parental consent: Yes. Youth athletes and a parent or guardian must sign a statement acknowledging receipt of the official concussion policy.

Immediate removal from play: Yes. Any athlete suspected of having sustained a concussion in a practice or game must be immediately removed from play.

Return-to-play guidelines and clearance: Concussed athletes must be evaluated by and receive written consent from a licensed health care provider with specific training in the evaluation and management of concussion before returning to play. Licensed health care providers must also indicate, in writing, that they have "successfully completed a continuing education course in the evaluation and management of concussion."

Application to private leagues: Yes. Extends to all amateur and youth leagues, both public and private, and to student athletes under age eighteen.

Vermont

SENATE BILL 100

SIGNED INTO LAW: MAY 2011

EFFECTIVE: START OF THE FALL 2011 ATHLETIC SEASON

Education: The commissioner of education, assisted by selected members of the Vermont Principals' Association, must develop statewide concussion guidelines to educate coaches, parents, and student athletes. Coaches must receive concussion identification and management training at least every two years.

Mandatory parental consent: Yes. Youth athletes and a parent or guardian must sign a statement acknowledging receipt of concussion-related educational materials on a yearly basis.

Immediate removal from play: No

Return-to-play guidelines and clearance: Concussed athletes must be evaluated by and receive written consent from a licensed health care provider with specific training in the evaluation and management of concussion before returning to play.

Application to private leagues: None

Virginia

SENATE BILL 652

SIGNED INTO LAW: APRIL 2010

EFFECTIVE: JULY 2011

Education: Calls for the board of education to develop and distribute concussion guidelines.

Mandatory parental consent: Yes. Youth athletes and a parent or guardian must sign a concussion and head injury information sheet on a yearly basis.

Immediate removal from play: Yes. Any athlete suspected of having sustained a concussion in a practice or game must be immediately removed from play and is barred from same-day return to play.

Return-to-play guidelines and clearance: Concussed athletes must be evaluated by and receive written consent from a licensed health care provider before returning to play.

Application to private leagues: None

Washington

HOUSE BILL 1824: "ZACKERY LYSTEDT LAW"

SIGNED INTO LAW: MAY 2009

EFFECTIVE: JULY 2009

Education: Calls for each school district's board of directors to work with the Washington Interscholastic Activities Association to develop concussion-management guidelines.

Mandatory parental consent: Yes. Youth athletes and a parent or guardian must sign a concussion and head injury information sheet on a yearly basis.

Immediate removal from play: Yes. Any athlete suspected of having sustained a concussion in a practice or game must be immediately removed from play.

Return-to-play guidelines and clearance: Concussed athletes must be evaluated by and receive written consent from a licensed health care provider with specific training in the evaluation and management of concussion before returning to play.

Application to private leagues: None

West Virginia

SENATE BILL 340

Status: Pending

Wisconsin

ASSEMBLY BILL 259

Status: Pending

Wyoming

SENATE FILE 38

SIGNED INTO LAW: MARCH 2011

EFFECTIVE: JULY 2011

Education: Calls for the state superintendent to assist local school districts in developing protocols to address the risks associated with concussions, yet specifically states that "no district shall be required to adopt any part of [these] protocols."

Mandatory parental consent: No

Immediate removal from play: No

Return-to-play guidelines and clearance: None

Application to private leagues: None

References

INTRODUCTION

1. Moser, R., Schatz, P., & Jordan, M. (2005). Prolonged effects of concussion in high school athletes. *Neurosurgery, 57*(2), 300–306.

2. Allen, K. Trying to keep a star on ice. *USA Today*, pp. E1–E2. October 8, 1998.

3. Concussions reported in NFL up 21 percent from last season. Associated Press. December 13, 2010. http://www.nfl.com/.

4. Schwarz, A. Ad change underlines influence of NFL. *New York Times*. January 21, 2011. http://www.nytimes.com/.

5. Leahy, S. After latest rule change, James Harrison says NFL officials 'are idiots.' *USA Today*. May 25, 2011. http://content.usatoday.com/.

6. Schwarz, A. Madden puts concussions in new light in his game. *New York Times*. April 2, 2011. http://www.nytimes.com/.

7. Rhoden, W. Some players see hypocrisy, not dirty hits. *New York Times*. December 3, 2010. http://www.nytimes.com/.

8. Allen, K. Sidney Crosby concussions raise questions about head-shot rule. *USA Today*. January 25, 2011. http://www.usatoday.com/.

9. Brooks, L. Rangers' Boogaard died from accidental overdose. *New York Post*. May 21, 2011. http://www.nypost.com/.

10. Garcia-Roberts, G. Dave Duerson's secret life and tragic end. *Miami New Times*. April 28, 2011. http://www.miaminewtimes.com/.

11. Walsh, N. Pro-bowler Dave Duerson's suicide renews head trauma debate. ABCNews.com. February 26, 2011. http://abcnews.go.com/.

12. Martland, H. (1928). Punch drunk. *JAMA, 91*(15), 1103–1107.

13. Laskas, J. Game brain. *GQ*. October 2009. http://www.gq.com/.

14. Loh, S. What Chris Henry taught us: How an autopsy of the former Cin-

cinnati Bengals' receiver's brain has helped doctors further research about concussions in football. *The Patriot-News.* August 22, 2010. http://blog.pennlive.com/.

15. Omalu, B., DeKosky, S., Minster, R., Kamboh, M., Hamilton, R., & Wecht, C. (2005). Chronic traumatic encephalopathy in a National Football League player. *Neurosurgery, 57*(1), 128–34.

16. McKee, A., Cantu, R., Nowinski, C., Hedley-White, E., Gavett, B., Budson, A., Santini, V., Lee, H., Kubilus, C., & Stern, R. (2009). Chronic traumatic encephalopathy in athletes: Progressive tauopathy after repetitive head injury. *Journal of Neuropathology and Experimental Neurology, 68*(7), 709–735.

17. Schwarz, A. Duerson's brain trauma diagnosed. *New York Times.* May 2, 2011. http://www.nytimes.com/.

18. Smith, S. Tests reveal former NFL player suffered from brain disease. CNN.com. May 2, 2011. http://www.cnn.com/.

19. Schwarz, A. Former Bengal Henry found to have had brain damage. *New York Times.* June 28, 2010. http://www.nytimes.com/.

20. Keating, P. Researchers find brain trauma in Henry. *ESPN The Magazine.* June 2010.

21. Schwarz, A. Suicide reveals signs of a disease seen in NFL. *New York Times.* September 13, 2010. http://www.nytimes.com/.

22. Dingfelder, S. Contact sports may put teens at risk for a rare degenerative brain disease. *Monitor on Psychology, 40*(5), 11. May 2009.

23. Walsh, N. Pro-bowl player's suicide renews head trauma debate. *MedPage Today.* February 25, 2011. http://www.medpagetoday.com/.

24. Brain expert: Kids shouldn't play contact sports. TheBostonChannel.com. September 13, 2011. http://www.thebostonchannel.com/.

25. Guskiewicz, K., McCrea, M., Marshall, S., Cantu, R., Randolph, C., Barr, W., Onate, J., & Kelly, J. (2003). Cumulative effects associated with recurrent concussion in collegiate football players: The NCAA concussion study. *JAMA, 290*(19), 2549–2555.

26. Shephard, R. (1997). Curricular physical activity and academic performance. *Pediatric Exercise Science, 9,* 113–125.

27. Tremblay, M., Inman, J., & Willms, J. (2000). The relationship between physical activity, self-esteem, and academic achievement in 12-year-old children. *Pediatric Exercise Science, 12,* 312–324.

28. Seefeldt, V., & Ewing, M. (1996). Youth sports in America: An overview. *PCPFS Research Digest, Series 2*(11), 19.

29. National Federation of High School Associations [NFHS]. (2006). *High School Athletics Participation Survey.* 2005–2006. Indianapolis, IN: NFHS. http://www.cdc.gov/mmwr/.

30. Bakhos, L., Lockhart, G., Myers, R., Linakis, J. (2010). Emergency department visits for concussion in young child athletes. *Pediatrics, 126*(3), e550–e556. Originally published online. Doi: 10.1542/peds.2009–3101.

31. Abel, D. Bill addressing student concussions advances. *Boston Globe.* April 28, 2010. http://www.boston.com/.

32. McCrea, M., Guskiewicz, K., Marshall, S., Barr, W., Randolph, C., Cantu, R., Onate, J., Yang, J., & Kelly, J. (2003). Acute effects and recovery time following concussion in collegiate football players: The NCAA concussion study. *JAMA, 290*(19), 2556–2563.

33. Cusimano, M. (2009). Canadian minor hockey participants' knowledge about concussion. *Canadian Journal of Neurological Science, 36*(3), 315–320.

34. Iverson, G., Lovell, M., & Smith, S. (2000). Does brief loss of consciousness affect cognitive functioning after mild head injury? *Archives of Clinical Neuropsychology, 15*(7), 643–648.

CHAPTER 1

1. Giza, C., & Hovda, D. (2001). The neurometabolic cascade of concussion. *Journal of Athletic Training, 36*(3), 228–325.

2. Gruber, H., & Voneche, J. (1977). The essential Piaget. New York: Basic Books.

3. Field, M., Collins, M., Lovell, M., & Maroon, J. (2003). Does age play a role in recovery from sports-related concussion? A comparison of high school and collegiate athletes. *Journal of Pediatrics, 142,* 546–553.

4. Delaney, J., Lacroix, V., Leclerc, S., & Johnston, K. (2002). Concussions among university football players and soccer players. *Clinical Journal of Sport Medicine, 12*(6), 331–338.

5. Colvin, A., Mullen, J., Lovell, M., West, R., Collins, M., & Groh, M. (2009). The role of concussion history and gender in recovery from soccer-related concussion. *American Journal of Sports Medicine, 37*(9), 1699–704.

6. Sokolove, M. The uneven playing field. *New York Times.* May 11, 2008. http://www.nytimes.com/.

7. Bäckström, T. Epileptic seizures in women related to plasma estrogen and progesterone during the menstrual cycle. (1976). *Acta Neurologica Scandinavica, 54*(4), 321–47.

8. McMahon, Patrick J. (2006). Current diagnosis and treatment in sports medicine. New York: McGraw-Hill Companies.

9. Haugh, D. Seattle-area teen helps NFL, others see dangers in concussions from football. *Chicago Tribune.* October 17, 2010. http://articles.chicagotribune .com/.

10. Centers for Disease Control and Prevention. (1997). Sports-related recurrent brain injuries–United States. *Morbidity and Mortality Weekly Report, 46*(10), 224–227.

11. Kelly, J., Rosenberg, J. (1997). The diagnosis and management of concussion in sports. *Neurology, 48,* 575–580.

12. Pellman, E., Viano, D., Tucker, A., Casson, I., Waeckerie, J. Concussion in professional football: reconstruction of game impacts and injuries. (2003). *Neurosurgery, 53*(4), 799–812.

13. Kluger, J. Headbanger nation. *Time.* February 3, 2011. http://www.time .com/.

14. Moser, R. Knock knock: Concussions from sports injuries. *New Jersey Medicine.* November 1998, 27–29.

15. Kozlowski, K., Leddy, J., Tomita, M., Bergen, A., & Willer, B. (2007). Use of the ICECI and ICE-10 E-coding structures to evaluate causes of head injury and concussion from sport and recreation participation in a school population. *NeuroRehabilitation, 22*(3), 191–198.

16. Epstein, D. Sports genes. *Sports Illustrated.* May 17, 2010. http://sports illustrated.cnn.com/vault/.

17. Jordan, B., Relkin, N., Ravdin, L., Jacobs, A., Bennett, A., & Gandy, S. Apolipoprotein E epsilon 4 associated with chronic traumatic brain injury in boxing. (1997). *JAMA 278*(2), 136–140.

18. Finder, C. Experts warn about repeated brain blows in football. *Pittsburgh Post-Gazette.* June 28, 2010. http://www.post-gazette.com/.

19. Stein, R. Genetic testing for sports genes courts controversy. *Washington Post.* May 18, 2011. http//:www.washingtonpost.com/national/.

20. Terrell, T., Bostick, R., Abramson, R., Xie, D., Barfield, W., Cantu, R., Stanek, M., & Ewing, T. (2008). APOE, APOE promoter, and tau genotypes and risk for concussion in college athletes. *Clinical Journal of Sport Medicine, 18*(1), 10–17.

21. Moser, R., Schatz, P. (2002). Enduring effects of concussions in young athletes. *Archives of Clinical Neuropsychology 17,* 91–100.

22. Schatz, P., Moser, R., Covassin, T., & Karpf, R. (2011). Early indicators of cognitive, emotional, and physical effects in high school athletes with multiple previous concussions. *Neurosurgery, 68*(6), 1562–1567.

23. Wolfley, B. Fox's Aikman takes a pass on concussion issue. *Milwaukee Journal Sentinel.* January 8, 2011. http://www.jsonline.com/blogs/sports/.

CHAPTER 2

1. McCrea, M., Kelly, J., Randolph, C., Kluge, J., Bartolic, E., Finn, G., & Baxter, B. (1998). Standardized assessment of concussion (SAC). *Journal of Head Trauma Rehabilitation, 13*(2), 27–35.

2. Barth, J., Alves, W., Ryan, T., Macciocchi, S., Rimel, R., Jane, J., & Nelson, W. (1989). Mild head injury in sports: Neuropsychological sequelae and recovery of function. In H. Levin, J. Eisenberg, & A. Benton (Eds.), *Mild Head Injury* (pp. 257–275). New York: Oxford University Press.

3. Quality Standards Subcommittee of the American Academy of Neurology. (1997). Practice parameter: The management of concussion in sports (summary statement). http://www.aan.com/.

4. Iverson, G., Lovell, M., & Smith, S. (2000). Does brief loss of consciousness affect cognitive functioning after mild head injury? *Archives of Clinical Neuropsychology, 15*(7), 643–648.

5. Guskiewicz, K., Weaver, N., Padua, D., & Garrett, W. (2000). Epidemiology of concussion in collegiate and high school football players. *American Journal of Sports Medicine, 28*(5), 643–650.

6. Lovell, M., Collins, M., Iverson, G., Field, M., Maroon, J., Cantu, R., Podell, K., Powell, J., Belza, M., & Fu, F. (2003). Recovery from mild concussions in high school students. *Journal of Neurosurgery, 98*(2), 296–301.

7. Aubry, M., Cantu, R., Dvorak, J., Graf-Baumann, T., Johnston, K., Kelly, J, Lovell, M., McCrory, P., Meeuwisse, W., & Schamasch, P. (2002) Summary and agreement statement of the 1st international symposium concussion in sport, Vienna. *Clinical Journal of Sport Medicine, 12*(1), 6–11.

8. Collins, M., Lovell, M., Maroon, J., Cantu, R., & McKeag, D. (2002). Memory dysfunction eight days post-concussion in high school athletes. *Medicine & Science in Sports & Exercise, 34*(5), S298.

9. Galetta, K., Barret, J., Allen, M., Madda, D., Delicata, A., Tennant, C., Branas, M., Maguire, L., Messner, S., Devick, S., & Balcer, L. (2011). The King-Devick test as a determinant of head trauma and concussion in boxers and MMA fighters. *Neurology 76*, 1456–1462.

10. Barton, Lindsay. King-Devick test promises more rapid, reliable sideline screening for concussions. Momsteam.com. February 16, 2011. http://www .momsteam.com/.

11. Lovell, M., Pardini, J., Welling, J., Collins, M., Bakal, J., Lazar, N., Roush, R., Eddy, W., & Becker, J. (2007). Functional brain abnormalities are related to clinical recovery and time to return-to-play in athletes. *Neurosurgery, 61*(2), 352–360.

12. Zoroya, G. 360,000 veterans may have brain injuries. *USA Today*. March 5, 2009. http://www.usatoday.com/.

13. Drummond, K. Billions of dollars later, military docs still can't spot brain injuries. Wired.com. June 8, 2010. http://www.wired.com/.

14. Miller, C., & Zwerdling, D. Military still failing to diagnose, treat brain injuries. NPR.org. June 8, 2010. http://www.npr.org/.

15. Banyan Biomarkers, Inc. awarded $26.3 million department of defense contract for diagnostic test for traumatic brain injury (press release). Businesswire .com. October 5, 2010. http://www.businesswire.com/.

16. Assael, S. Blood simple: on-field tests could soon take the guesswork out of identifying concussions. *ESPN The Magazine*. January 6, 2011. http://sports .espn.go.com/nfl/.

17. McCrea, M., Hammeke, T., Olsen, G., Leo, P., & Guskiewicz, K. (2004). Unreported concussion in high school football players: Implications for prevention. *Clinical Journal of Sport Medicine, 14*(1), 13–17.

CHAPTER 3

1. Barth, J., Alves, W., Ryan, T., Macciocchi, S., Rimel, R., Jane, J., & Nelson, W. (1989). Mild head injury in sports: Neuropsychological sequelae and recovery of function. In H. Levin, H. Eisenberg, & A. Benton (Eds.), *Mild Head Injury* (pp. 257–275). New York: Oxford University Press.

2. Kluger, J. Headbanger nation. *Time*. February 3, 2011. http://www.time .com/.

3. Moser, R., Charlton-Fryer, A., & Berardinelli, S. (2010). Youth and sports concussion: A heads up on the growing public health concern. In F. Webbe (Ed.), *Handbook of Sport Neuropsychology*. New York: Springer Publishing Company.

4. Lovell, M. ImPACT Version 6.0 Clinical User's Manual. (2007). http://www .impacttest.com/.

5. Schatz, P., Moser, R., Solomon, G., Ott, S., & Karpf, R. (in press). Incidence of invalid computerized baseline neurocognitive test results in high school and college students. *Journal of Athletic Training*.

6. Suhr, J., & Gunstad, J. (2002). "Diagnosis threat": The effect of negative expectations on cognitive performance in head injury. *Journal of Clinical and Experimental Neuropsychology, 24*(4), 448–457.

7. Moss, A., Jones, C., Fokias, D., & Quinn, D. (2003). The mediating effects of effort upon the relationship between head injury severity and cognitive functioning. *Brain Injury, 17*(5), 377–387.

8. Lovell, M., Collins, M., Maroon, J., Cantu, R., Hawn, M., Burke, C., & Fu, F. (2002). Inaccuracy of symptom reporting following concussion in athletes. *Medicine & Science in Sports & Exercise*, 34(5), S298.

9. McCrea, M., Hammeke, T., Olsen, G., Leo, P., & Guskiewicz, K. (2004). Unreported concussion in high school football players: implications for prevention. *Clinical Journal of Sport Medicine*, 14(1), 13–17.

10. Bailey, C., & Arnett, P. (2006). Motivation and the assessment of sports-related concussion. In S. Slobounov & W. Sebastianelli (Eds.), *Foundation of Sports-Related Concussion* (pp. 171–193). New York: Springer Publishing Company.

11. Schatz, P., Neidzwski, K., Moser, R., & Karpf, R. (2010). Relationship between subjective test feedback provided by high-school athletes during computer-based assessment of baseline cognitive functioning and self-reported symptoms. *Archives of Clinical Neuropsychology*, 25(4), 285–292.

12. Green, P., Iverson, G., & Allen, L. (1999). Detecting malingering in head injury litigation with the word memory test. *Brain Injury*, 13(10), 813–819.

13. Green, P., Rohling, M., Lees-Haley, P., & Allen, L. (2001). Effort has a greater effect on test scores than severe brain injury in compensation claimants. *Brain Injury*, 15(12), 1045–1060.

14. Schatz, P., Pardini, J., Lovell, M., Collins, M., & Podell, K. (2006). Sensitivity and specificity of the ImPACT test battery for concussion in athletes. *Archives of Clinical Neuropsychology*, 21(1), 91–99.

15. Schatz, P. (2009). Long-term test-retest reliability of baseline cognitive assessments using ImPACT. *American Journal of Sports Medicine*, 38(1), 47–53.

16. Schatz, P., Moser, R., Solomon, G., Ott, S., & Karpf, R. (in press). Incidence of invalid computerized baseline neurocognitive test results. *Journal of Athletic Training*.

17. Covassin, T., Elbin, R., & Stiller-Ostrowski, J. (2009). Current sport-related concussion teaching and clinical practices of sports medicine professionals. *Journal of Athletic Training*, 44(4), 400–404.

18. Preidt, R. Validity of baseline concussion tests questioned. *USA Today*. June 17, 2011. http://www.usatoday.com/.

19. UT Arlington researcher tests reliability of popular concussion measurement tool (press release). University of Texas at Arlington. June 24, 2011.

CHAPTER 4

1. Lovell, M., Pardini, J., Welling, J., Collins, M., Bakal, J., Lazar, N., Roush, R., Eddy, W., & Becker, J. (2007). Functional brain abnormalities are related to clinical recovery and time to return-to-play in athletes. *Neurosurgery, 61*(2), 352–360.

2. Abel, D. Bill addressing student concussions advances. *Boston Globe.* April 28, 2010. http://www.boston.com/news/education/.

3. Colombo, J., Kannass, K., Shaddy, J., Kundurthi, S., Maikranz, J., Anderson, C., Blaga, O., & Carlson, S. (2004). Maternal DHA and the development of attention in infancy and toddlerhood. *Child Development, 75*(4),1254–1267.

4. University of Georgia Athletic Association. Concussion management guidelines. May 30, 2010. http://www.ncaa.org/.

5. Oz, M. Playing Defense. *Time.* February 3, 2011. http://www.time.com/.

6. Stones, M. US military may 'shock and awe' omega-3 market. Nutraingredients-usa.com. February 2, 2010. http://www.nutraingredients-usa.com/.

7. Shah, S. Military deploys acupuncture to treat soldiers' concussions. McClatchy Newspapers. February 7, 2011. http://www.mcclatchydc.com/.

8. Barton, L. More post-concussion help for students in classroom needed. Momsteam.com. April 24, 2011. http://www.momsteam.com/.

CHAPTER 5

1. Finder, C. Former football player's concussion has altered his life. *Pittsburgh Post-Gazette.* January 2, 2011. http://www.post-gazette.com/.

2. Plevretes, Preston. Second impact syndrome (interview). ESPN.com. http://search.espn.go.com/preston-plevretes/.

3. Genuardi, F., & King, W. (1995). Inappropriate discharge instructions for youth athletes hospitalized for concussion. *Pediatrics, 95*(2), 216–218.

4. Bazarian, J., Veenema, T., Brayer, A., & Lee, E. (2001). Knowledge of concussion guidelines among practitioners caring for children. *Clinical Pediatrics*, *40*(4), 201–212.

5. Yang, J., Phillips, G., Xiang, H., Allareddy, V., Heiden, E., & Peek-Asa, C. (2008). Hospitalisations for sport-related concussion in US children aged 5 to 18 years during 2000–2004. *British Journal of Sports Medicine*, *42*(8), 664–669.

6. McCrory, P., Meeuwisse, W., Johnston, K., Dovrak, J., Aubry, M., Molloy, M., & Cantu, R. (2009). Consensus statement on concussion in sport—the 3rd international conference on concussion in sport, held in Zurich, November 2008. *Journal of Clinical Neuroscience*, *16*, 755–763.

7. Maugans, T., Farley, C., Mekibib, A., Leach, J., & Cecil, K. (2012). Pediatric sports-related concussion produces cerebral blood flow alterations. *Pediatrics*, *129*(1), 28–37.

8. Schwarz, A. Overseers vow to work on standards for helmets. *New York Times*. January 24, 2011. http://query.nytimes.com/.

9. Schwarz, A. Soon, helmet data at a keystroke. *New York Times*. January 8, 2011. http://www.nytimes.com/.

10. Virginia Tech National Impact Database. May 2011. http://www.sbes.vt.edu/nid.php

11. Schwarz, A. Researchers employ new test to estimate concussion risk for helmets. *New York Times*. May 10, 2011. http://www.nytimes.com/.

12. De Lench, B. Concussion bill of rights #7: A safe helmet for every child. Momsteam.com. http://www.momsteam.com/.

13. Schwarz, A. Group to phase out old football helmets. *New York Times*. March 10, 2011. http://www.nytimes.com/.

14. Dorsey, P. Helmet tech aimed at concussions. ESPN.com. September 1, 2009. http://sports.espn.go.com/ncaa/.

15. See the Xenith website at http://www.xenith.com/football/one-player-one-helmet/.

16. Mihalik, J., McCaffrey, M., Rivera, E., Pardini, J., Guskiewicz, K., Collins, M., & Lovell, M. (2007) Effectiveness of mouthguards in reducing neurocog-

nitive deficits following sports-related cerebral concussion. *Dental Traumatology, 23*(1), 14–20.

17. Benson, B., Hamilton, G., Meeuwisse, W., McCrory, P., Dvorak, J. (2009). Is protective equipment useful in preventing concussion? A systematic review of the literature. *British Journal of Sports Medicine, 43(Suppl 1),* i56–67.

18. Daneshvar, D., Baugh, C., Nowinski, C., McKee, A., Stern, R., & Cantu, R. (2011). Helmets and mouth guards: the role of personal equipment in preventing sport-related concussion. *Clinical Journal of Sport Medicine, 30*(1), 145–63.

19. Moser, R., Schatz, P., & Jordan, B. (2005). Prolonged effects of concussion in high school athletes. *Neurosurgery, 57*(2), 300–306.

20. Schatz, P., Moser, R., Covassin, T., & Karpf, R. (2011) Early indicators of enduring symptoms in high school athletes with multiple previous concussions. *Neurosurgery, 68*(6), 1562–1567.

21. Gessel, L., Fields, S., Collins, C., Dick, R., & Comstock, R. (2007). Concussion among United States high school and collegiate athletes. *Journal of Athletic Training, 42*(4), 495–503.

22. Schatz, P. & Moser, R. (2011). Current issues in pediatric sports concussion. *The Clinical Neuropsychologist, 25,* 1042–1057.

23. McCrory, P., Meeuwisse, W., Johnston, K., Dovrak, J., Aubry, M., Molloy, M., & Cantu, R. (2009). Consensus statement on concussion in sport—the 3rd international conference on concussion in sport, held in Zurich, November 2008. *Journal of Clinical Neuroscience, 16,* 755–765.

CHAPTER 6

1. C. S. Mott Children's Hospital. C. S. Mott Children's Hospital national poll on children's health. Ann Arbor: University of Michigan Department of Pediatrics and Communicable Diseases, and the University of Michigan Child Heath Evaluation and Research (CHEAR) Unit. Vol. 10.1. June 14, 2010.

2. Athletic trainers fill a necessary niche in secondary schools (news release). National Association of Athletic Trainers. March 12, 2009. http://www.nata.org/NR031209.

3. Schools adjust to new N.C. concussion law. *StarNewsOnline*. July 2, 2011. http://www.starnewsonline.com/.

4. Moser, R., Glatts, C., & Schatz, P. (in review). Efficacy of immediate and delayed cognitive and physical rest following sports-related concussion.

5. Engh, F. (1999). *Why Johnny Hates Sports: Why Organized Youth Sports Are Failing Our Children and What We Can Do about It* (p. 73). New York: Avery.

CHAPTER 7

1. Hayes, A., & Martinez, M. Former NFL players: League concealed concussion risks. CNN.com. July 20, 2011. http://www.cnn.com/.

2. Fleming, C. NFL's headaches continue . . . for brain injuries. PacificNorthwest InjuryLawAdvocate.com. July 25, 2011. http://www.pacificnorthwestinjury lawadvocate.com/.

3. Habib, H. Mark Duper, O.J. Anderson among 75 retirees suing NFL over concussions. *Palm Beach Post*. July 20, 2011. http://www.palmbeachpost.com/.

4. Laskas, J. Game brain. *GQ*. October 2009. http://www.gq.com/.

5. Culhane, J. Concussions and cigarettes: A new lawsuit claims the NFL is like big tobacco. Does the case have merit? Slate.com. July 26, 2011. http://www .slate.com/.

6. Pellman, E., & Viano, D. (2006). Concussion in professional football: summary of the research conducted by the National Football League's committee on mild traumatic brain injury. *Neurosurgical Focus, 21*(4), E12.

7. '88 plan': Honor for a declining NFL warrior. Associated Press. March 23, 2007. http://nbcsports.msnbc.com/.

8. Mihoces, G. NFL begins debate about concussions at summit. *USA Today*. June 20, 2007. http://www.usatoday.com/.

9. Davis, G. NFL finally paying greater heed to concussion risks . . . with low-quality poster. Sportsgrid.com. July 27, 2010. http://www.sportsgrid.com/nfl/.

10. NFL outlines for players steps taken to address concussions (press release). National Football League. Aug. 14, 2007. http://www.nfl.com/.

11. Schwarz, A. NFL issues new guidelines on concussions. *New York Times.* December 2, 2009. http://www.nytimes.com/.

12. Concussion: A must read for NFL players. Let's take brain injuries out of play (poster). Centers for Disease Control and Prevention. 2010. http://www.cdc.gov/.

13. Schwarz, A. In NFL fight, women lead the way. *New York Times.* April 10, 2010. http://www.nytimes.com/.

14. Henderson, J. Hall of famer Mackey leaves great legacy. TampaBayOnline.com. July 9, 2011. http://www2.tbo.com/.

15. Schwarz, A. N.F.L. picks new chairmen for panel on concussions. *New York Times.* March 16, 2010. http://www.nytimes.com/.

16. Nack, W. The wrecking yard. *Sports Illustrated.* May 7, 2001. http://www.sportsillustrated.com/.

17. Eichelberger, C. Ivy league schools are limiting football practices to reduce head injuries. Bloomberg.com. July 20, 2011. http://www.bloomberg.com/news/.

18. Klein, J. Hockey urged to ban all blows to the head by concussions panel. *New York Times.* October 20, 2010. http://www.nytimes.com/.

19. Klein, J. & Hackel, S. Researchers evaluate who is old enough for body checks. *New York Times.* February 5, 2011. http://slapshot.blogs.nytimes.com/.

20. Rodriguez, M. Proposed bodycheck ban stirs debate in youth hockey. BuffaloNews.com. June 6, 2011. http://www.buffalonews.com/sports/.

21. Silver, M. Inside the helmet: Eight of the NFL's most opinionated veterans talk exclusively, and candidly, with *GQ* about concussions, hard knocks, and the new rules of play. GQ.com. February 1, 2011. http://www.gq.com/sports/.

22. Gregory, S. The problem with football: How to make it safe. *Time.* January 28, 2010. http://www.time.com/.

23. Augustoviz, R. Checking ban for peewee hockey has governing bodies at odds. *StarTribune.* June 8, 2011. http://www.startribune.com/sports/.

24. Barton, L. Youth sports concussion safety laws: Idaho. Momsteam.com. March 31, 2011. http://www.momsteam.com.

25. Hurst, D. Plan to get tough on concussions stalls in committee over legal concerns. IdahoReporter.com. March 18, 2010. http://www.idahoreporter.com/.

26. Schwarz, A. A case against helmets in Lacrosse. *New York Times*. February 16, 2011. http://www.nytimes.com/.

27. Schwarz, A. Teaching young players a safer way to tackle. *New York Times*. December 25, 2010. http://www.nytimes.com/.

28. National SAFE KIDS Campaign, the National Athletic Trainers' Association and Johnson & Johnson. (2000). *Get into the Game: A National Survey of Parents' Knowledge, Attitudes, and Self-Reported Behaviors Concerning Sports Safety.* http://www.safekids.org/.

29. Moser, R., Charlton-Fryer, A., & Berardinelli, S. (2010). Youth and sports concussion: A heads up on the growing public health concern. In F. Webbe (Ed.), *Handbook of Sport Neuropsychology*. New York: Springer Publishing Company.

APPENDIX B

1. Guskiewicz, K., Weaver, N., Padua, D., & Garrett, W. (2000). Epidemiology of concussion in collegiate and high school football players. *American Journal of Sports Medicine, 28*(5), 643–650.

2. McKeever, C., & Schatz, P. (2003). Current issues in the identification, assessment, and management of concussion in sports-related injuries. *Applied Neuropsychology, 10*(1), 4–11.

3. Collins, M., Lovell, M., Maroon, J., Cantu, F., & McKeag, D. (2002). Memory dysfunction eight days post-concussion in high school athletes. *Medicine & Science in Sports & Exercise, 34,* 5.

4. Lovell, M., Pardini, J., Welling, J., Collins, M., Bakal, J., Lazar, N., Roush, R., Eddy, W., & Becker, J. (2007). Functional brain abnormalities are related to clinical recovery and time to return-to-play in athletes. *Neurosurgery, 61*(2), 352–360.

Index